# 1,000,000 Books

are available to read at

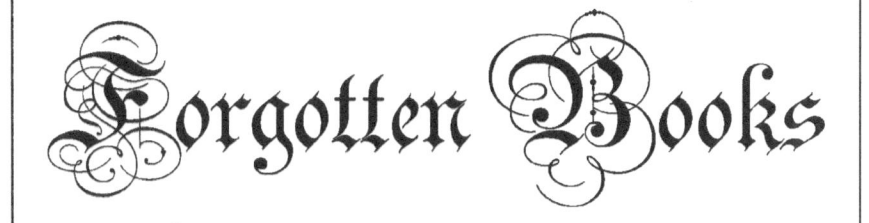

# Forgotten Books

www.ForgottenBooks.com

Read online
Download PDF
Purchase in print

ISBN 978-0-260-25376-7
PIBN 11011333

This book is a reproduction of an important historical work. Forgotten Books uses state-of-the-art technology to digitally reconstruct the work, preserving the original format whilst repairing imperfections present in the aged copy. In rare cases, an imperfection in the original, such as a blemish or missing page, may be replicated in our edition. We do, however, repair the vast majority of imperfections successfully; any imperfections that remain are intentionally left to preserve the state of such historical works.

Forgotten Books is a registered trademark of FB &c Ltd.
Copyright © 2018 FB &c Ltd.
FB &c Ltd, Dalton House, 60 Windsor Avenue, London, SW19 2RR.
Company number 08720141. Registered in England and Wales.

For support please visit www.forgottenbooks.com

# 1 MONTH OF FREE READING

at

www.ForgottenBooks.com

---

By purchasing this book you are eligible for one month membership to ForgottenBooks.com, giving you unlimited access to our entire collection of over 1,000,000 titles via our web site and mobile apps.

To claim your free month visit: www.forgottenbooks.com/free1011333

\* Offer is valid for 45 days from date of purchase. Terms and conditions apply.

English
Français
Deutsche
Italiano
Español
Português

# www.forgottenbooks.com

**Mythology** Photography **Fiction**
Fishing Christianity **Art** Cooking
Essays Buddhism Freemasonry
Medicine **Biology** Music **Ancient Egypt** Evolution Carpentry Physics
Dance Geology **Mathematics** Fitness
Shakespeare **Folklore** Yoga Marketing
**Confidence** Immortality Biographies
Poetry **Psychology** Witchcraft
Electronics Chemistry History **Law**
Accounting **Philosophy** Anthropology
Alchemy Drama Quantum Mechanics
Atheism Sexual Health **Ancient History**
**Entrepreneurship** Languages Sport
Paleontology Needlework Islam
**Metaphysics** Investment Archaeology
Parenting Statistics Criminology
**Motivational**

# Espy's Embalmer,

WITH NEARLY SEVENTY-FIVE CUTS AND
INSTRUCTIONS UNDER EACH CUT.

⚜

By J. B. Espy.

⚜

THE CUTS ARE REPRODUCTIONS OF PHOTOGRAPHS
TAKEN OF THE INSTRUMENTS IN THE HANDS OF
THE OPERATOR WHILE EMBALMING A DEAD BODY.

⚜

The Espy Fluid Company,
Publishers.

COPYRIGHT, APRIL 22, 1895.

W A

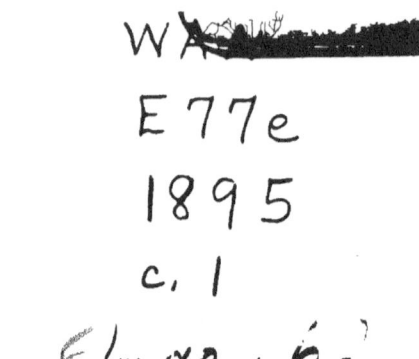

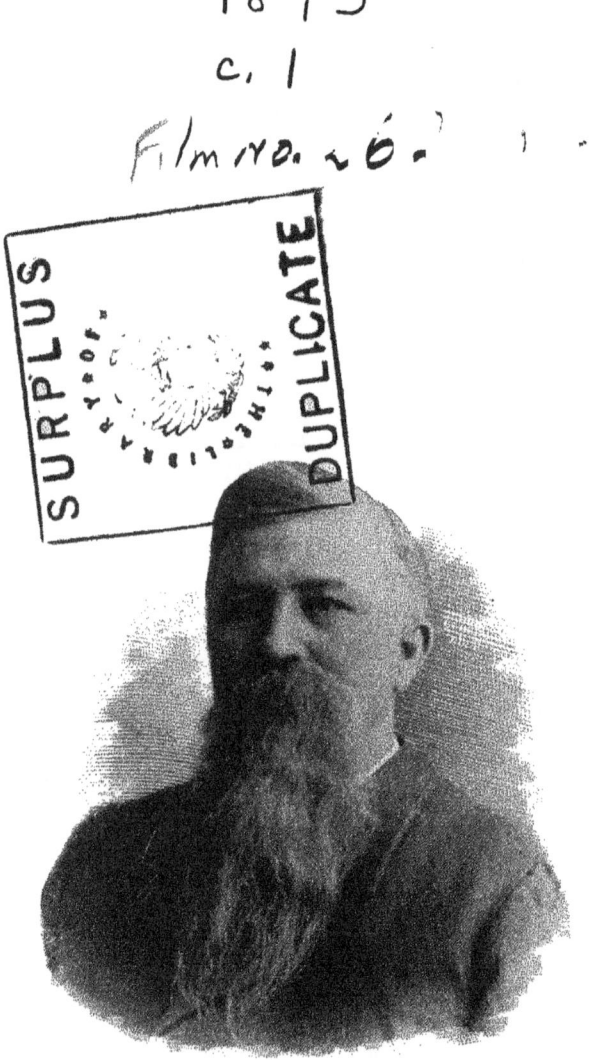

E77e
1895
c. 1

Film no. 6.

SURPLUS DUPLICATE

YOURS VERY TRULY

J. B. ESPY

# INTRODUCTION.

IN PREPARING this work on Embalming, for the Profession, the chief object has been to make it plain and easily understood. With this object in view, we have prepared cuts, reproductions of photographs, taken during the various operations in embalming a body. In the production of these cuts great care has been used to illustrate almost every turn of the instrument, while lifting the various arteries and veins in common use by the Profession.

The instructions accompanying each cut are in plain language, so as to be easily understood by everyone. The work also contains descriptions of the various and most successful ways of embalming the dead.

The Author does not pretend to be a Professor, but one, who by years of actual experience, has learned how to successfully embalm and preserve the dead.

We would have you remember that the first and most important step toward successful embalming, is to use a good fluid. This need will be met by using Espy's Embalming Fluid, which is "Excelled by None" as a disinfectant and preservative. There is no fluid on the market that has withstood such severe tests as Espy's Fluid. It can be used in the cavities, arteries or both.

In conclusion, we wish to say that we hope to have met at least some of the requirements of the Profession of the United States. We believe that if the Funeral Director, no matter how inexperienced he may be, will follow the instructions herein contained, he cannot fail doing his work correctly and obtaining the best results.

Respectfully yours,

THE ESPY FLUID CO.

## The Manner in Which to Proceed.

WHEN you are called upon to take charge of a dead body, first ascertain the cause of death and the condition of the body; by this you can decide how to proceed, for no person can make fixed rules by which one can be guided at all times. In ordinary cases, where there is no contagious disease, the following directions may help you:

First wet your hands in the fluid, or anoint them with Espy's Antiseptic Cream. If the case is a man, fill the rectum with cotton, and either draw the urine from the bladder with a No. 9 or a No. 12 Catheter or tie a string around the penis. (But if the case is a lady, have a very heavy diaper used.) Then lay the body on the board, ALWAYS at an incline.

The only way to properly embalm a body is to inject the entire vascular system. In some cases (in regard to which instructions will be found in the following pages) it is necessary to inject the cavities.

When you inject the whole vascular system, it is not necessary to use a bleacher, except in extremely bad cases. When you inject the cavities only, it is best to use a good bleacher, or the fluid diluted from one-half to three fourths, with water (per instructions on the following pages.)

Before dressing the body for the casket always sponge the face and hands with luke-warm water (except in dropsical cases.)

## Circulation of the Blood.

THE impure blood collects in the right auricle of the heart, which contracts slightly and forces the blood through the tri-cuspid valve into the right ventricle. The right ventricle contracts and forces the blood past the semi-lunar valve into the pulmonary artery. The tri-cuspid valve is closed by blood getting between its flaps and the wall of the heart and thus prevents the blood from going back into the right auricle. The pulmonary artery divides, sending off a branch to each lung. In the capillaries of the air-cells of the lungs, the blood is purified, giving up its carbonic acid gas and organic impurities, and receiving in return oxygen.

The blood then returns to the heart through the four pulmonary veins and enters the left auricle, which contracts slightly and forces the blood through the bi-cuspid valve into the left ventricle. The left ventricle contracts and forces the blood past the semi-lunar valves into the great aorta, the main trunk of the arterial system. The bi-cuspid valve closes like the tri-cuspid valve to prevent the blood from returning to the left auricle. The great aorta makes a bold curve, giving off branches to the head and arms, and then runs down the back of the chest, dividing and subdividing until it reaches every part of the body. The arteries at last end in the capillaries, where the blood is robbed of its oxygen and receives carbonic acid gas and organic impurities. It then returns through the veins, which unite and form the ascending and descending venæ cavæ that empty into the right auricle.

### Circulation of the Fluid in Arterial Embalming.

WHEN injecting embalming fluid into any of the four arteries given in the following pages, viz.: the radial, brachial, carotid or femoral; the fluid is forced up the artery (contrary to the course of the blood in life) to the aorta. Here, being prevented by the semi-lunar valves from entering the left side of the heart, it goes through the aorta and all its branches, until it reaches the capillaries. Passing through them it enters the venous system and returns to the right auricle through the ascending and descending venæ cavæ. It then passes down through the tri-cuspid valve into the right ventricle and out past the semi-lunar valve into the pulmonary artery; thence into the lungs. After permeating them, it returns to the left auricle, through the four pulmonary veins and then drops down into the left ventricle.

## How to Distinguish Arteries, Veins and Nerves.

The arteries are of a light color, and when you take hold of them they feel like, and have the appearance of a piece of rubber tubing. You may sometimes find blood in the arteries; when this is the case they are of a dark color, like the veins, but they can be distinguished from the veins, for when you take hold of a vein it feels thin and flat. The veins are always of a dark color and from one to three of them accompany each artery.

The nerves are always of a light color, and when you take hold of them they feel hard and round like a cord. The medium nerve crosses the brachial artery, about the middle of the arm, between the elbow and the shoulder.

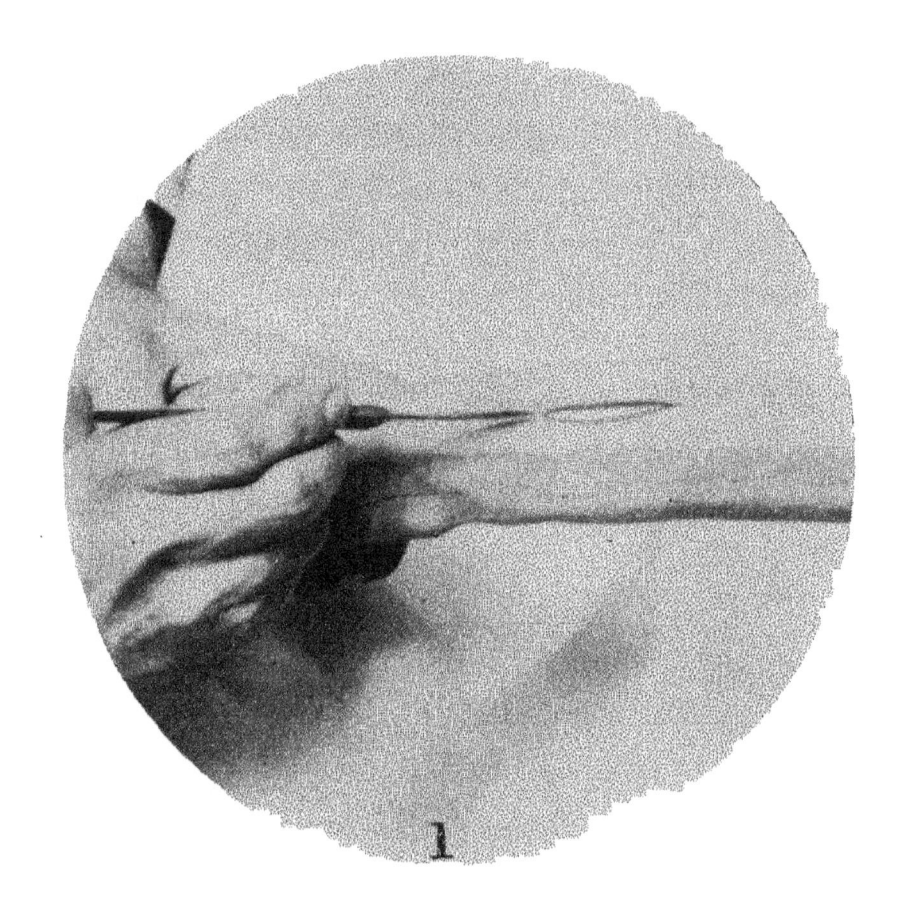

## TO RAISE THE RADIAL ARTERY.

The radial artery is the artery in which the pulse can be felt in life; it lies along the valley of the thumb side of the fore-arm, from the wrist to the elbow.

To raise this artery, take the scalpel and make an incision from three-quarters to one and a quarter inches long, just through the skin (as per cut).

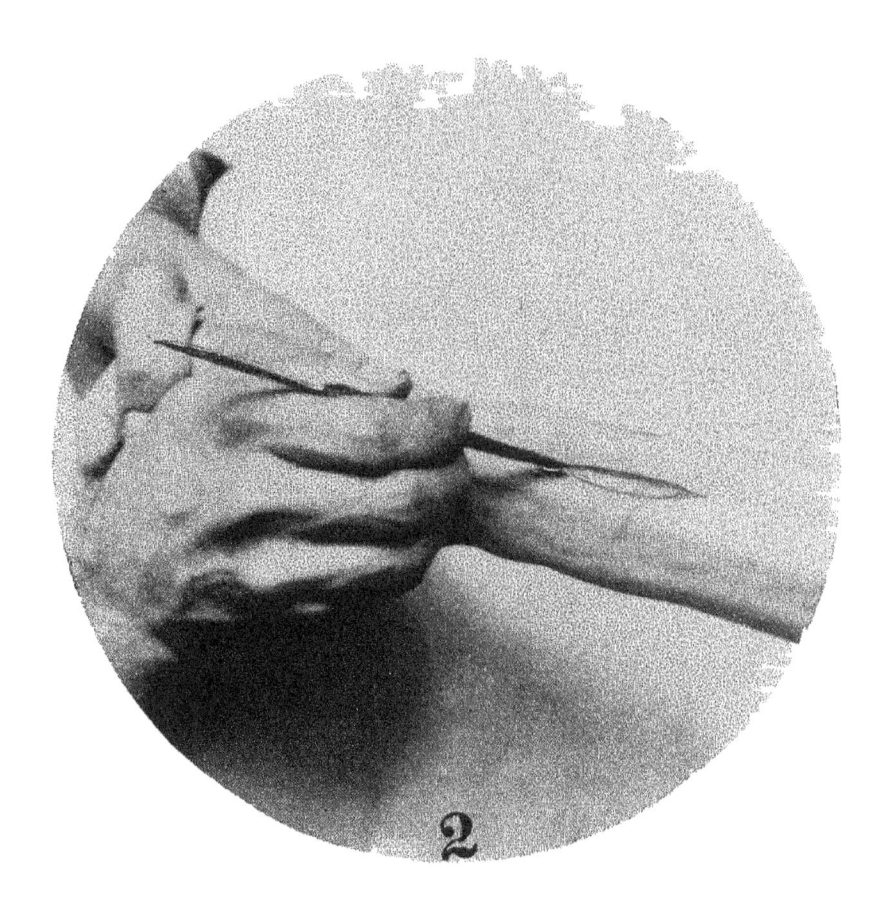

Now take the handle end of the scalpel, or aneurism needle, and work down through the fatty substance, to the deep fascia (as per cut).

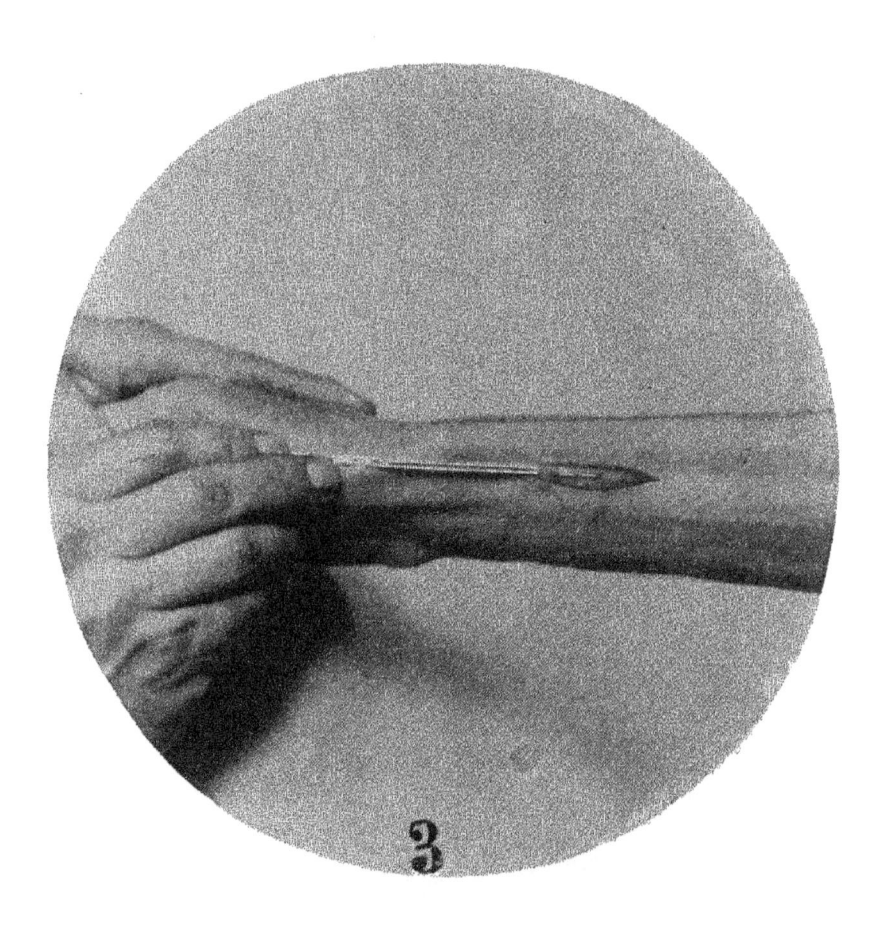

Next, take the sharp end of the fascia needle and puncture the deep fascia, at the lower end of the incision; then reverse the needle, enter the puncture, and run up under the deep fascia, with the groove of the needle up (as per cut).

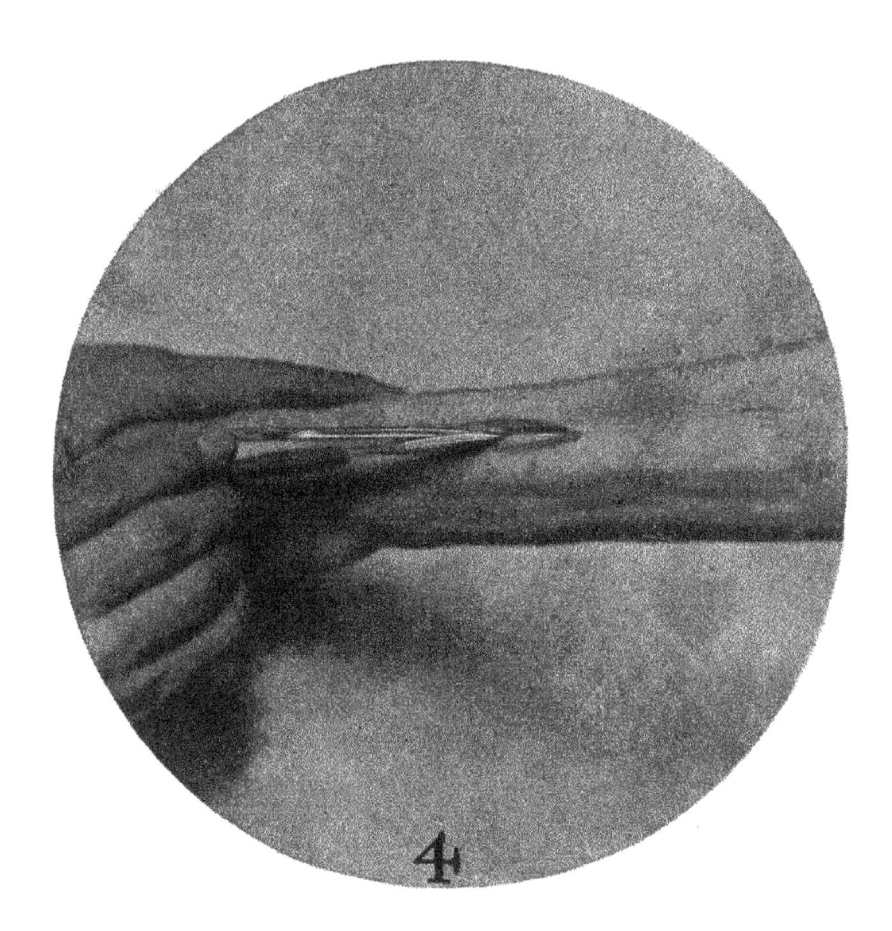

Then take the scalpel, lay its back in the groove of the fascia needle, and rip the deep fascia, the length of the incision (as per cut).

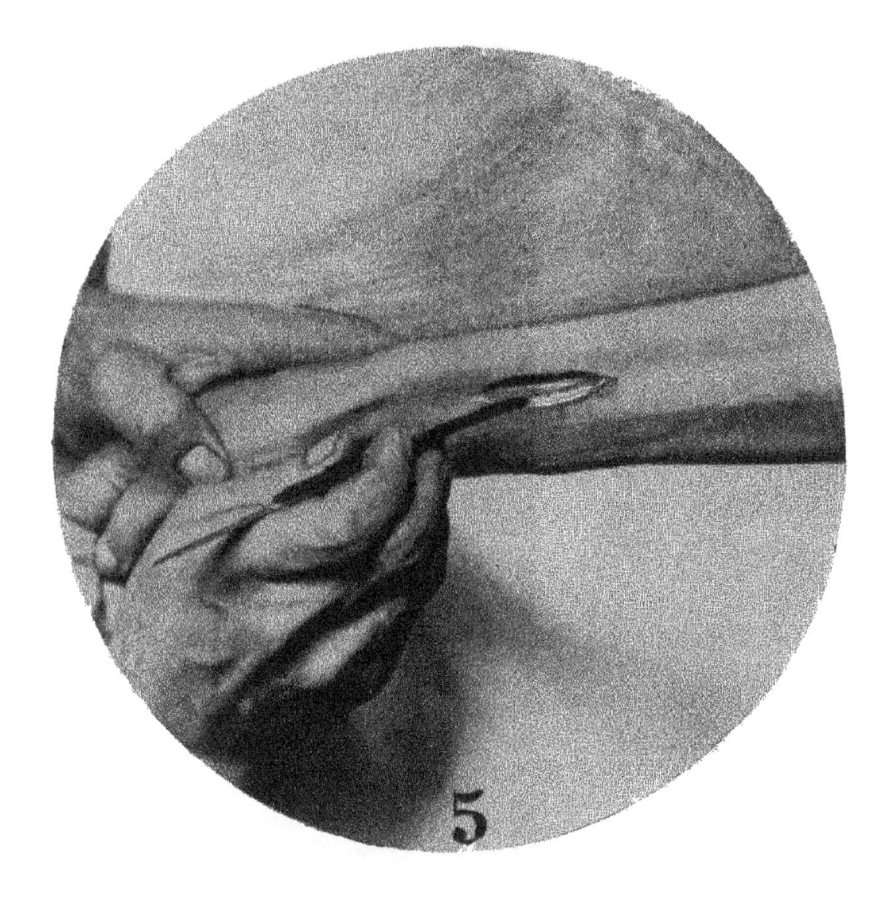

Take the aneurism needle or scalpel (as per cut), and work down through the fatty substance on both sides of the sheath containing the artery and vein.

## 6

Now take the aneurism needle, raise the sheath containing the artery and vein, and place the forceps under the artery (as per cut).

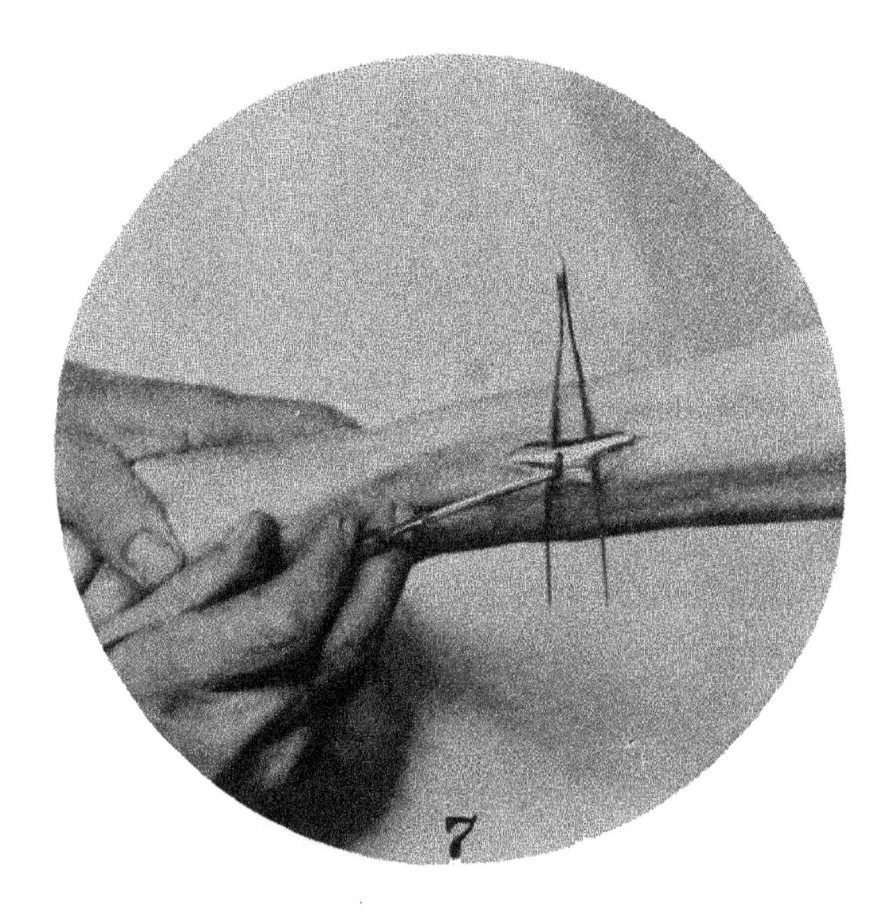

Now take the aneurism needle, and scratch along on the top of the sheath, to open it (as per cut).

## ESPY'S EMBALMER. 15

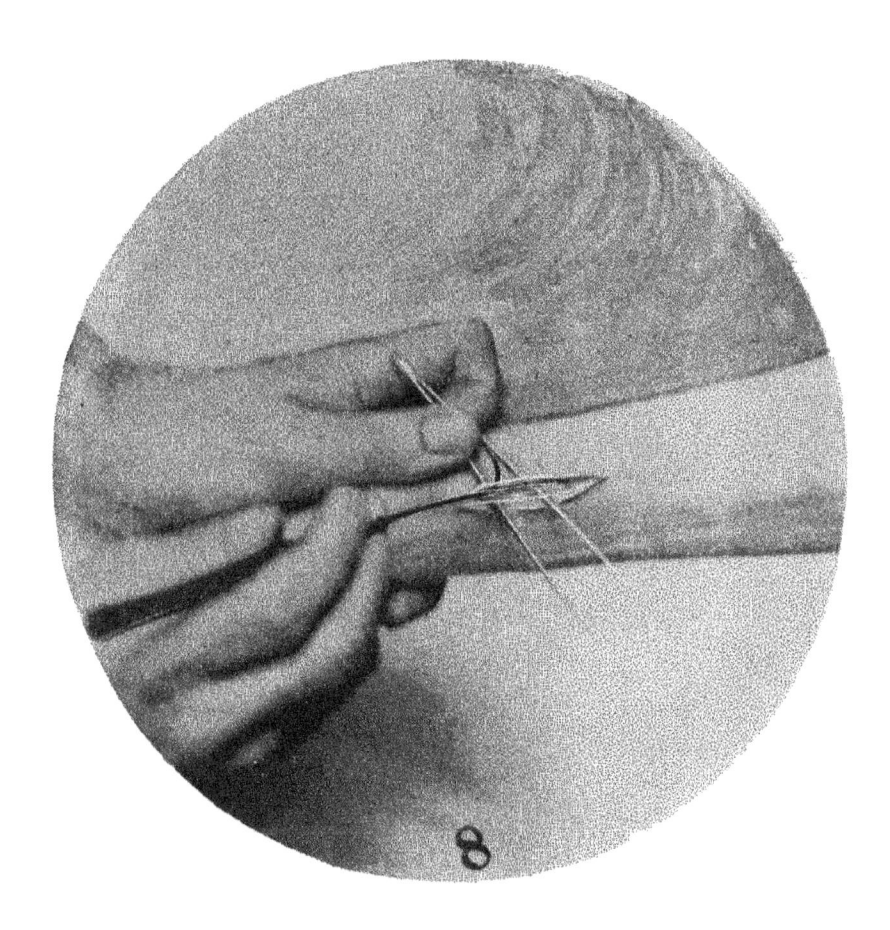

Then take the aneurism needle, lift the artery from out the sheath, and let the sheath and vein drop (as per cut); now place the forceps under the artery.

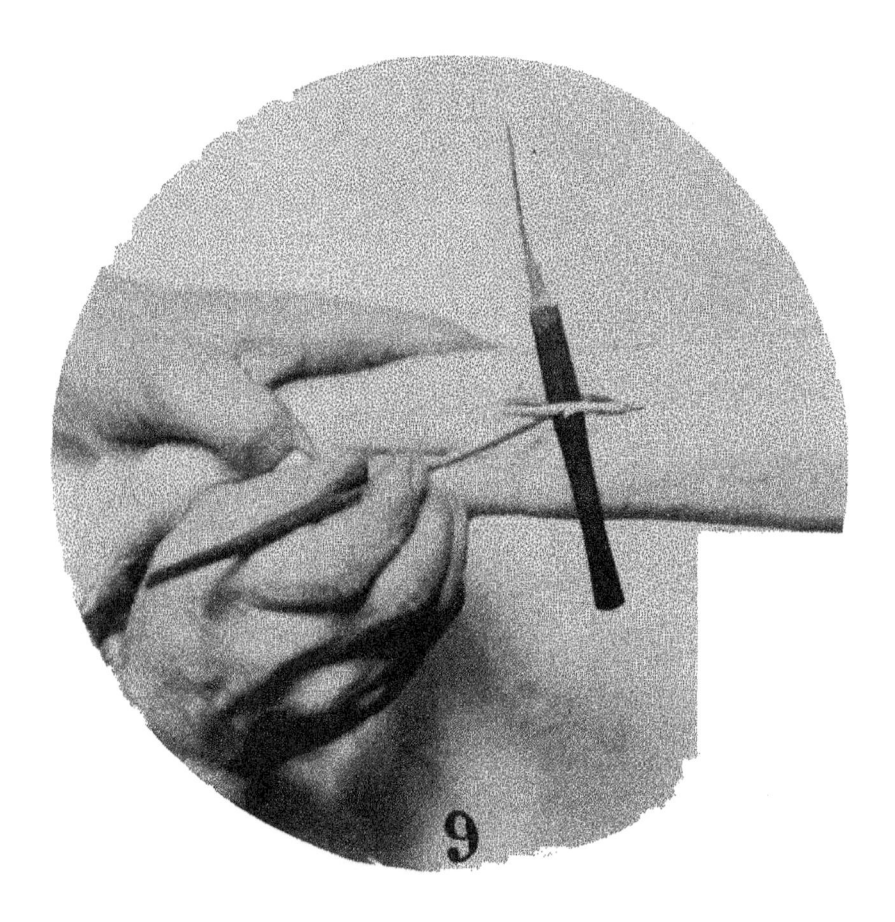

Now place the handle of the anuerism needle under the artery, and take out the forceps; then take the scalpel and nick the artery (as per cut).

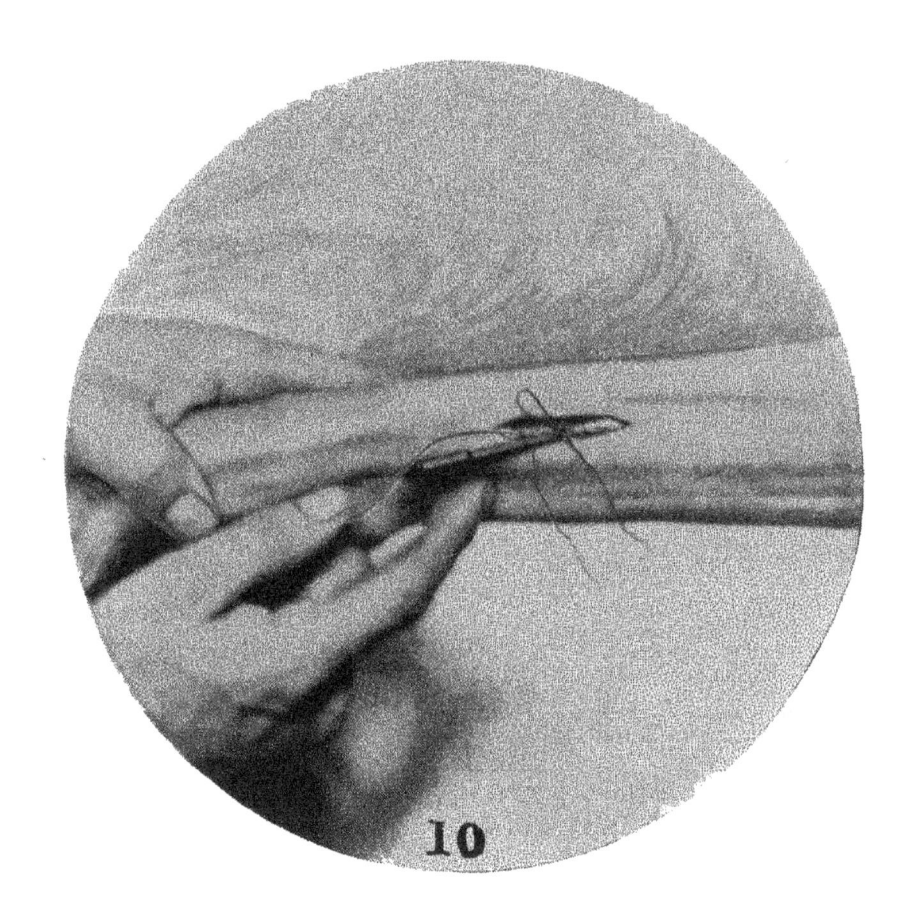

Next take two pieces of waxed thread, and place one at each end of the incision, under the artery; then take the small arterial tube and place it in the artery. Tie one hard knot and one bow knot behind the shoulder of the tube. Tie the other thread loosely around the artery (as per cut), until the fluid makes its appearance, while you are injecting the body; then tie it tightly.

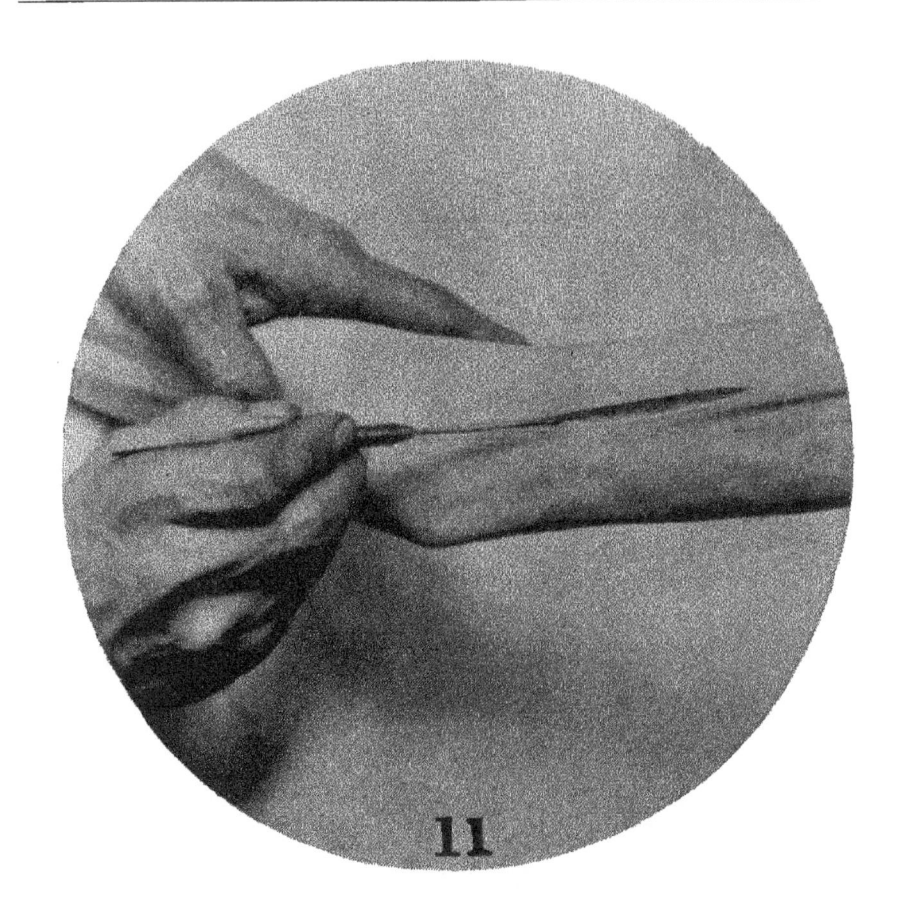

## TO RAISE THE BRACHIAL ARTERY.

To locate the brachial artery, trace the inner and under border of the biceps muscle, where you will always find the medium nerve, which crosses the brachial artery, about the center of the arm. The artery in the middle and lower third will follow the border of the muscle.

There are two ways of holding the arm while raising the brachial artery. One way is to lay the arm on your lap, take the scalpel and make an incision, just through the skin, from one and a half to two and a half inches long.

The other way is as follows: If operating upon the right arm (as per cut) place the right hand, *palm upwards*, in your left arm-pit, holding it securely between your arm and body. Then take the scalpel and make an incision, as above.

If you are left-handed and operating upon the left arm of the subject, place the left hand of the subject in you right arm-pit, holding it as the right arm.

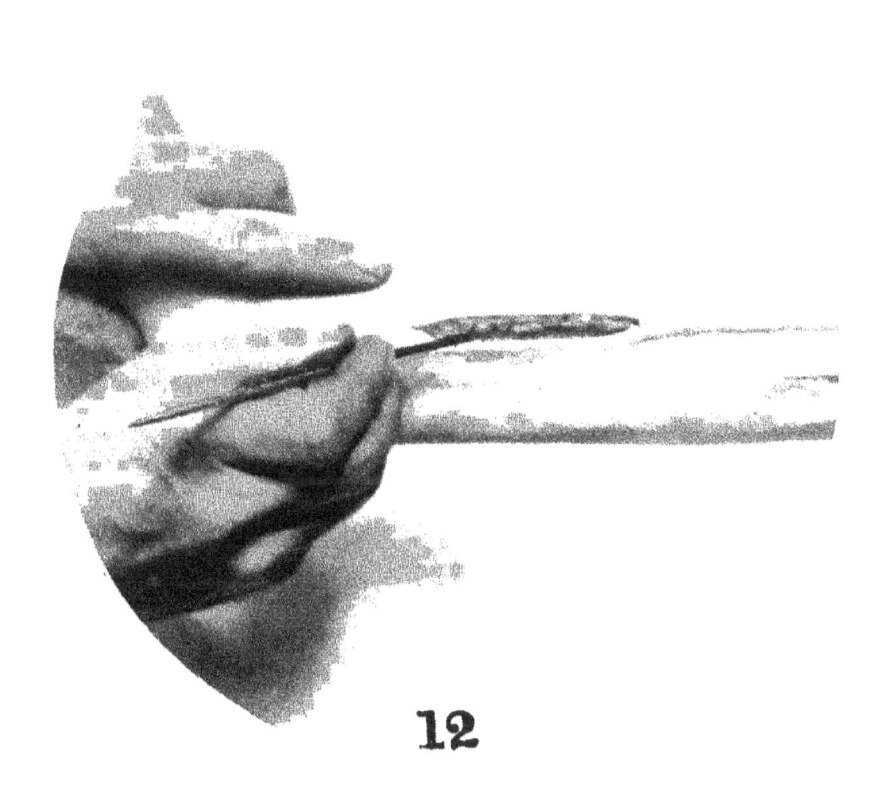

**12**

Now take the handle end of the scalpel or anuerism needle and work down through the fatty substance (as per cut). Underlying this, you will find the deep fascia.

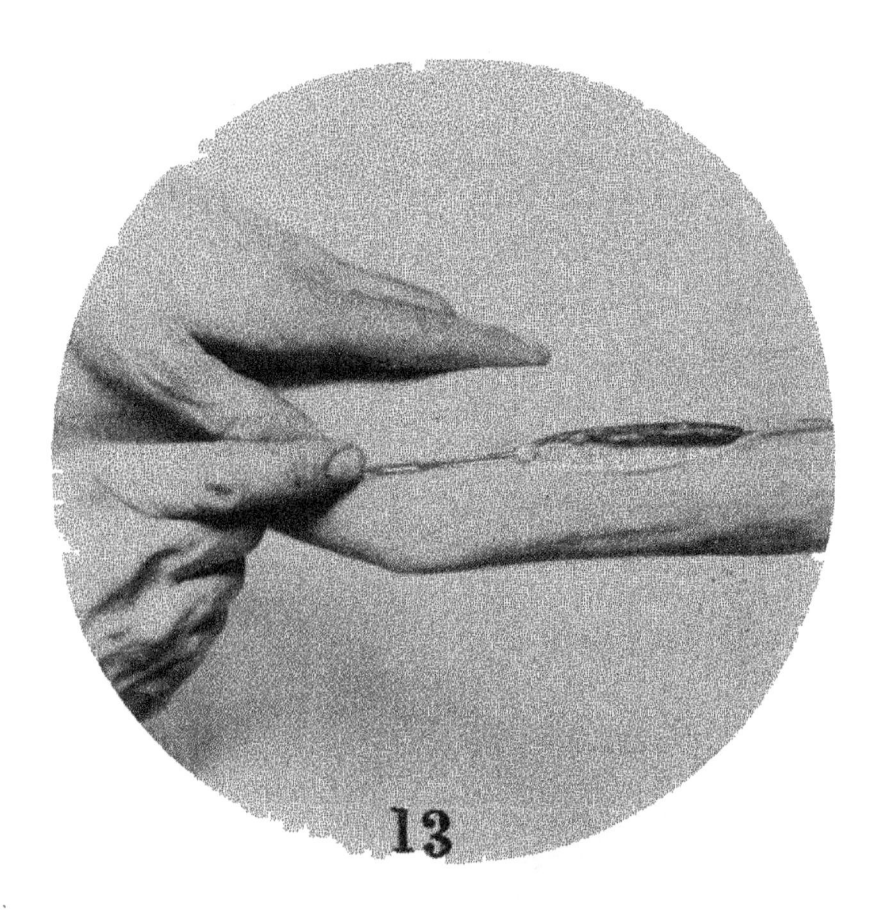

Next take the sharp end of the fascia needle, and puncture the deep fascia at the lower end of the incision; reverse the needle and run it up under the deep fascia, with the groove of the needle up (as per cut).

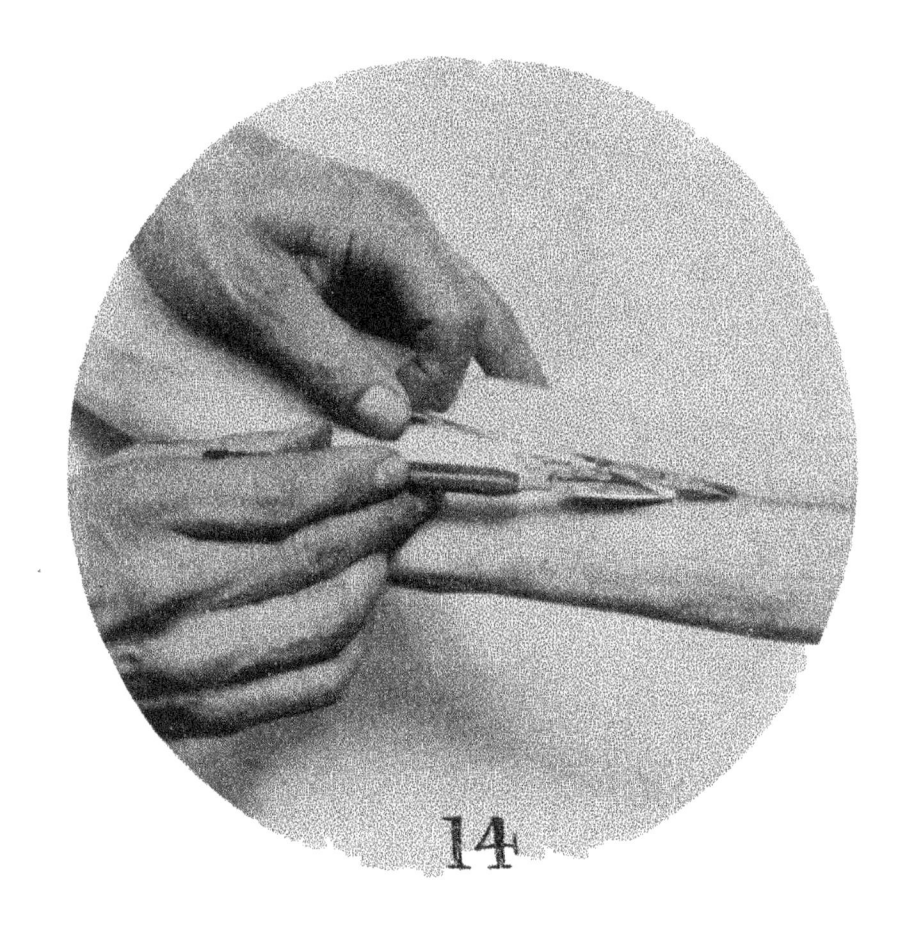

Take the scalpel, lay its back in the groove of the fascia needle and rip the deep fascia, the length of the incision (as per cut).

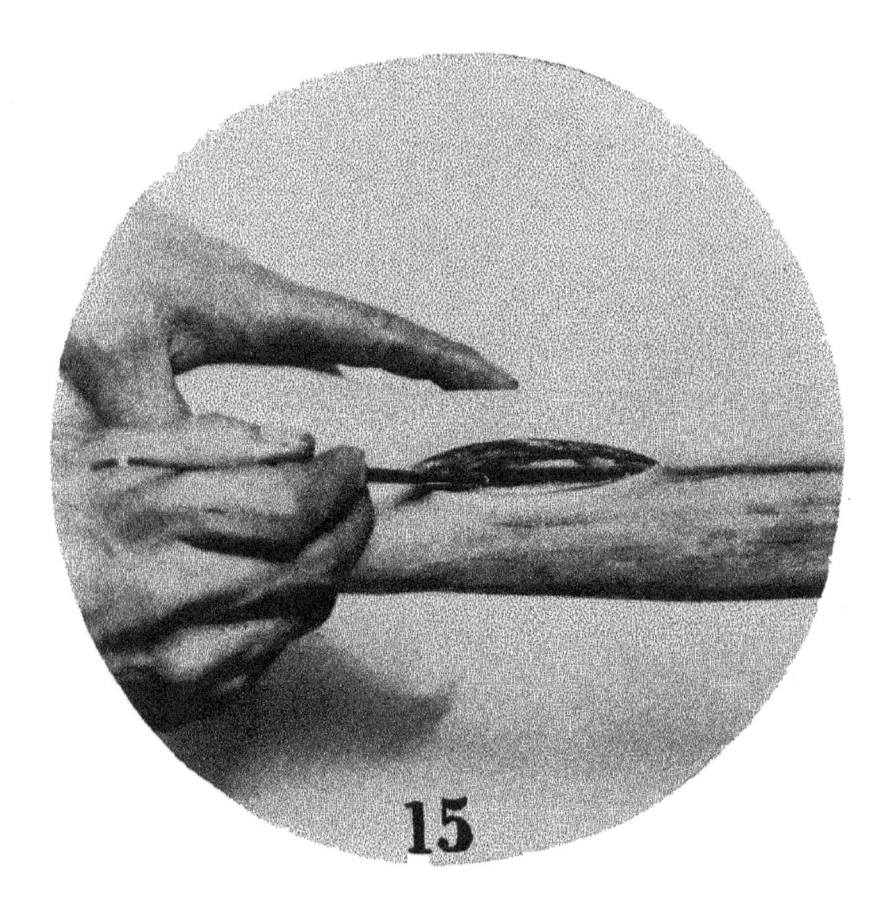

Now take the handle of the aneurism needle or scalpel and work down through the fatty substance, to the artery. Then work on down, separating the artery from the muscle on the one side, and from the nerve on the other side (as per cut).

16

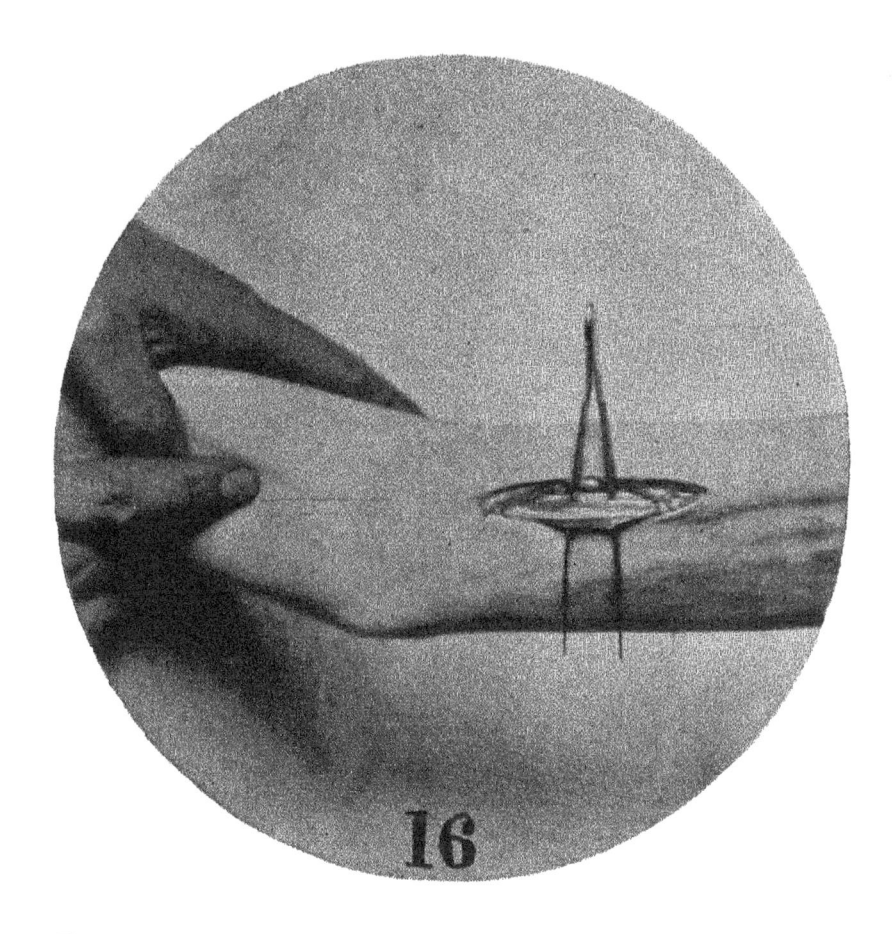

Take the aneurism needle, raise the artery and two veins, (which are all enclosed in the sheath) and place the forceps under as per cut).

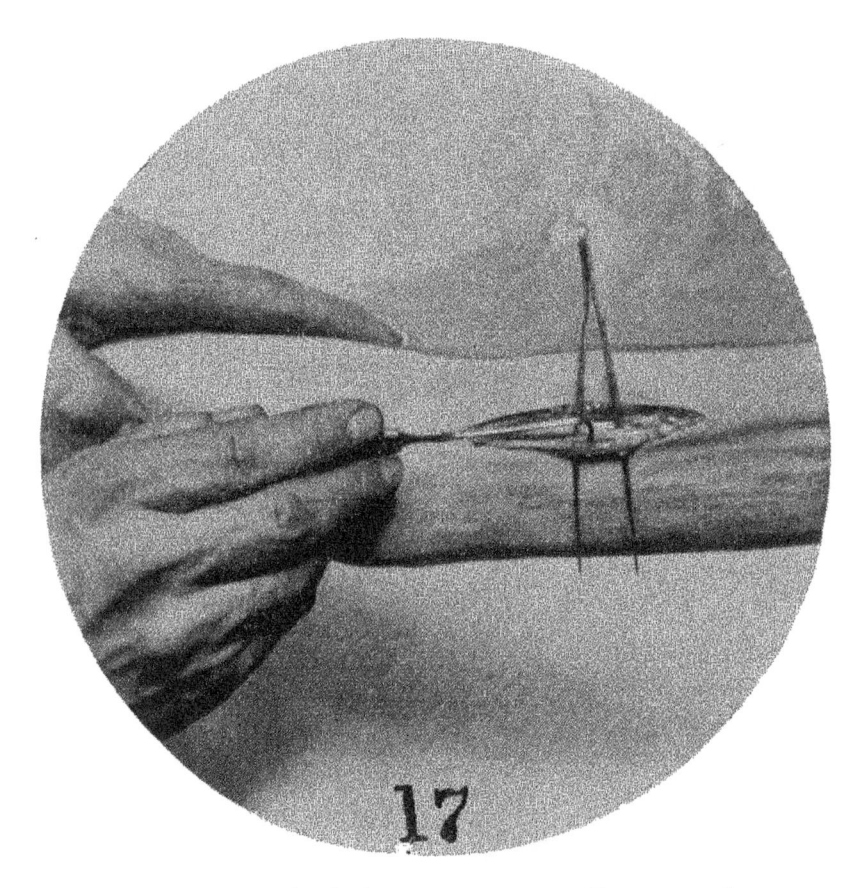

Take the hook-end of the aneurism needle, scratch on top of the sheath that surrounds the artery and two veins, to open it, (as per cut).

18.

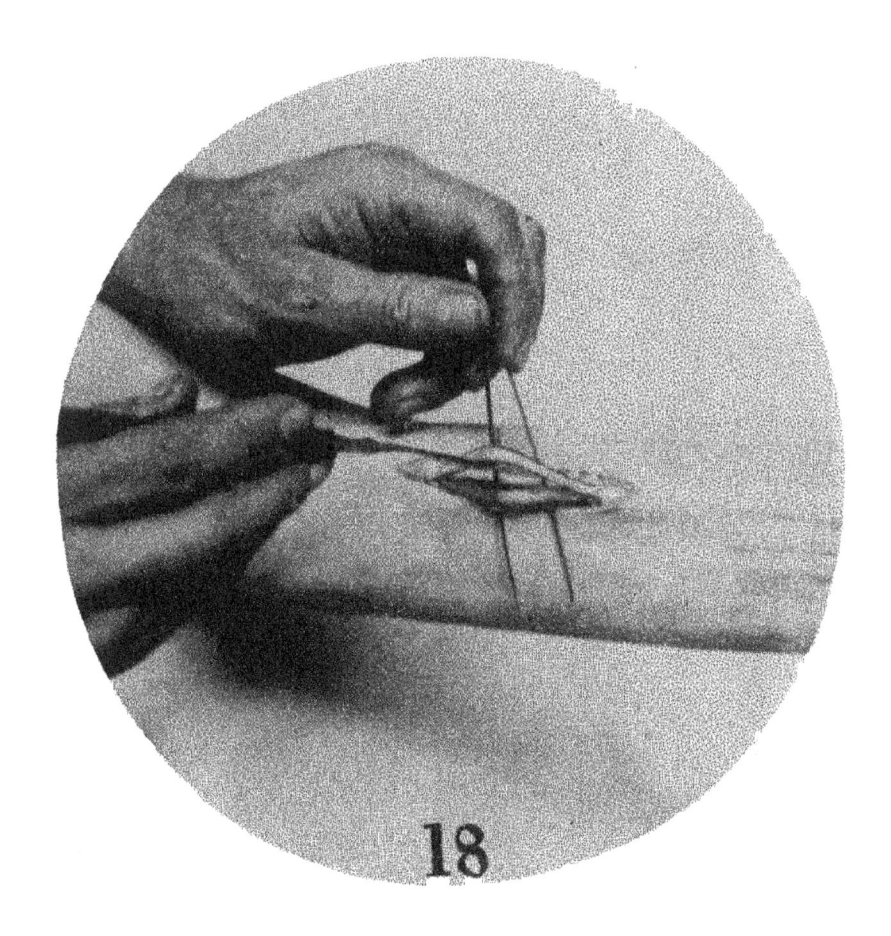

You will find the artery on top, the larger vein on the inner side and the smaller one underneath, the artery being of a lighter color than the veins, while the walls of the artery are thicker, resembling a piece of rubber tubing.

Take the hook end of the aneurism needle, put it under the artery and let the veins and sheath drop (as per cut). Then place the forceps under the artery.

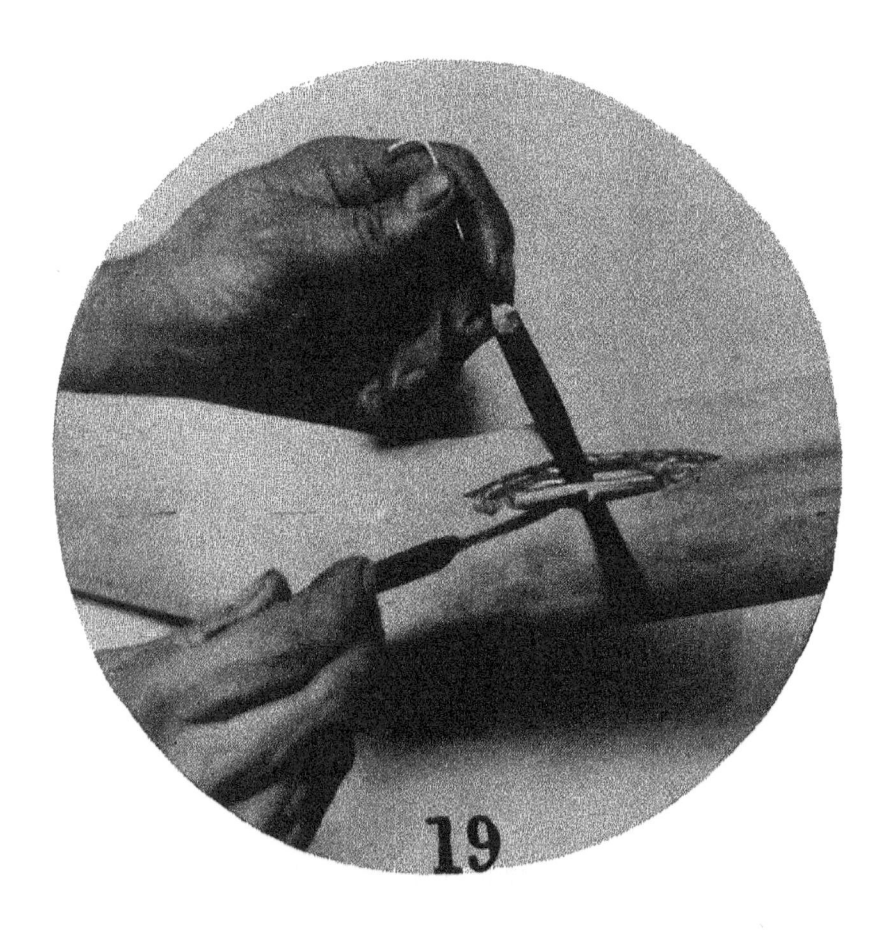

Now take the handle end of the aneurism needle, place it under the artery, and pull the forceps out. Then take the scalpel and nick the artery (as per cut).

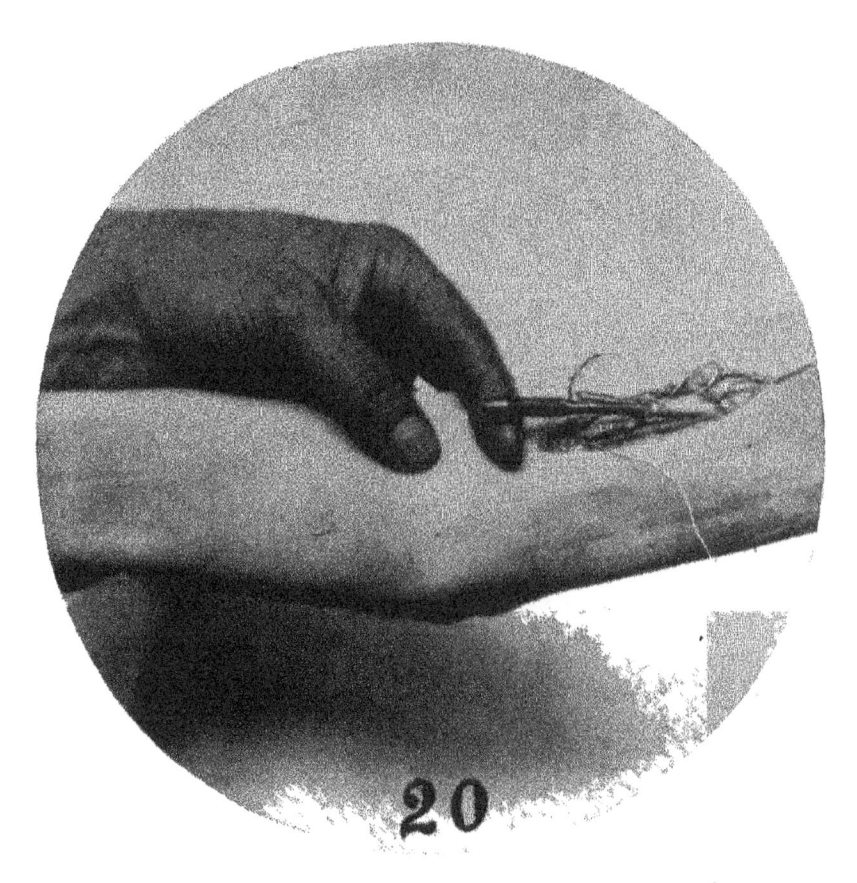

Next take two pieces of waxed thread, and put one at each end of the incision, under the artery; take the arterial tube and place it in the artery. Tie one hard knot and one bow knot behind the shoulder of the tube. Tie the other thread loosely around the artery (as per cut) until the fluid makes its appearance, while you are injecting the body; then tie tightly.

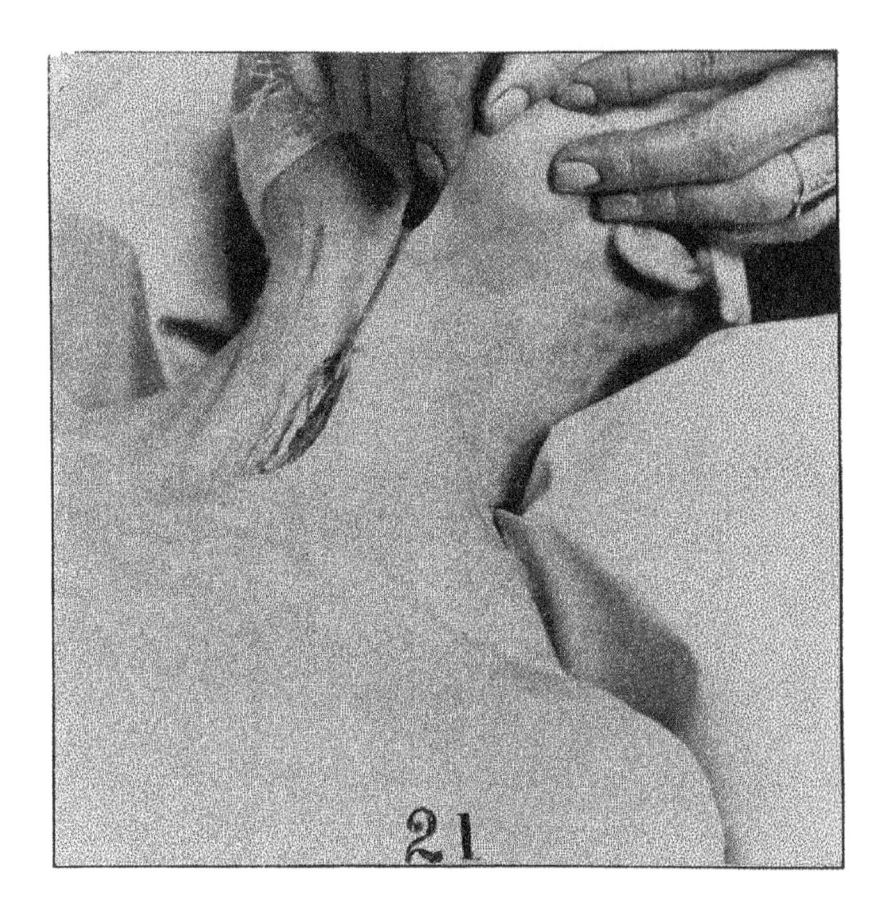

## TO LOCATE AND RAISE THE COMMON CAROTID ARTERY.
### PERPENDICULAR INCISION.

Stand at the head of the subject, raise the chin, pull the skin up and with the fingers trace the valley just outside the windpipe.

Use the scalpel and cut through the skin and thin sheet of muscle, known as the Platysma, commencing about one-half inch above the sternum or breast bone, and make the incision from two to two and one-half inches up, (as per cut).

Underneath this will be found, on the outer side, the Sternomastoid muscle, and on the inner side the Thyroid gland.

22

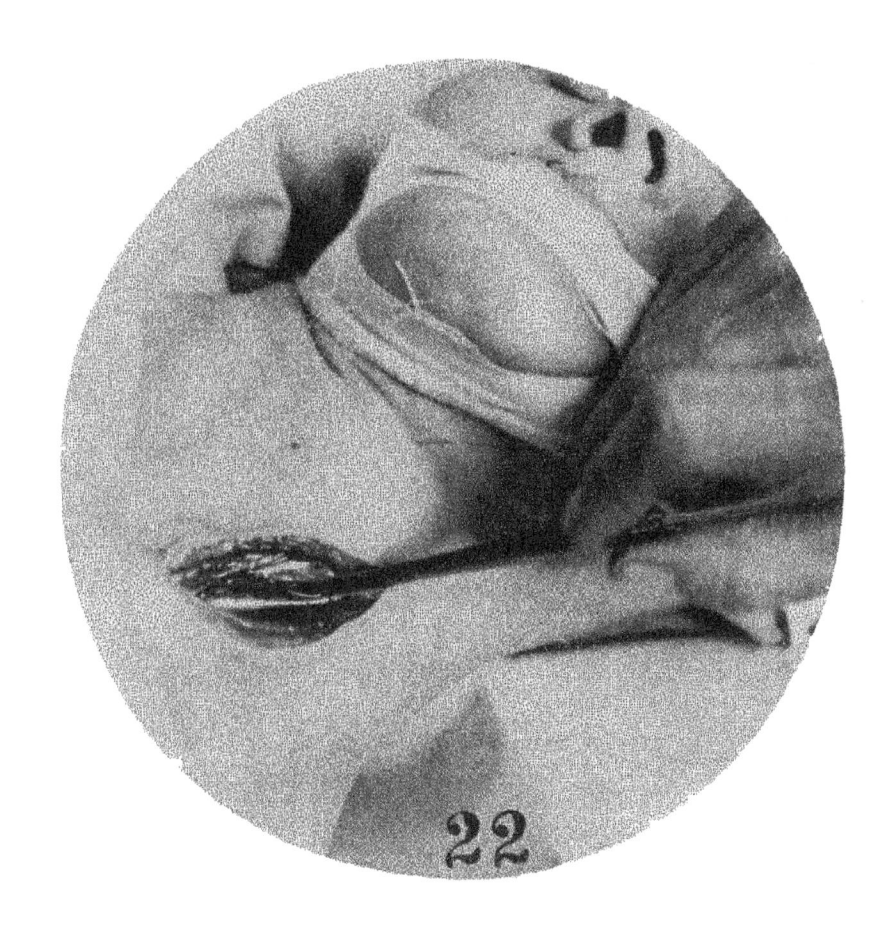

Now take the handle of the aneurism needle or scalpel and separate the Sternomastoid muscle from the Thyroid gland, which may be from one to one and one-half inches deep. Underneath these you will find the deep fascia, which may be split with the handle of the aneurism needle or scalpel (as per cut).

23

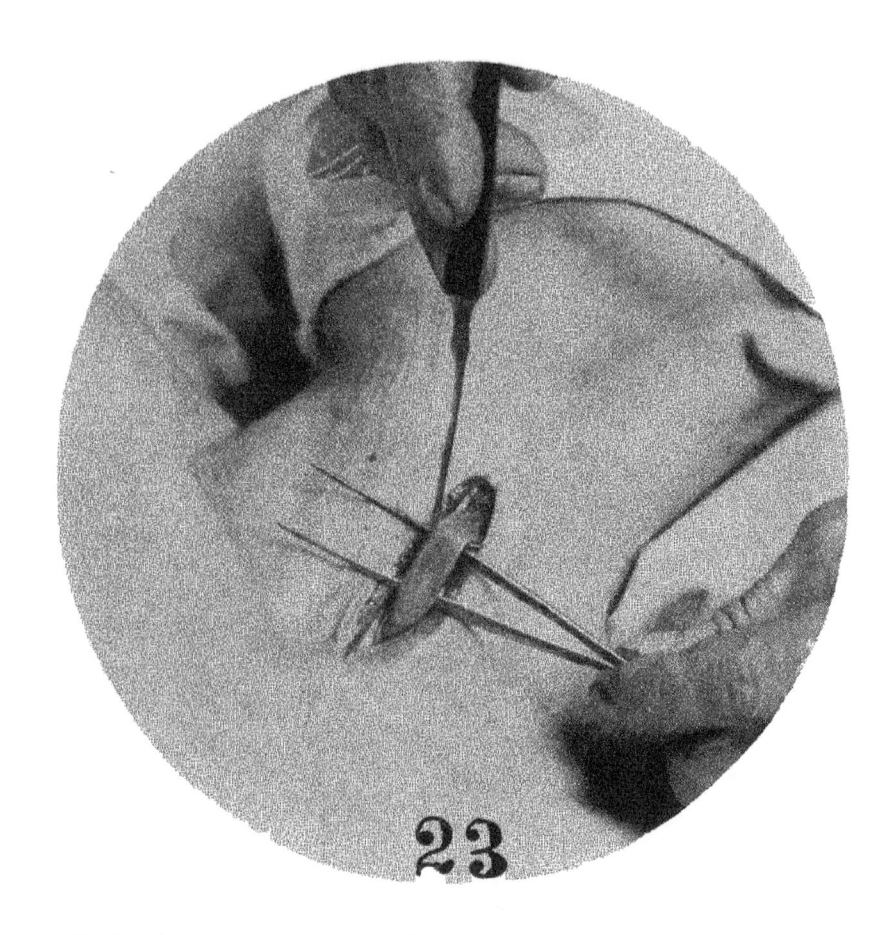

Hold the wound open and you may see the artery next the wind-pipe, and the vein on the outer side, both covered with a common sheath, which you can open by using the hook of the aneurism needle and tearing the sheath from off the artery, but not the vein. Then with the handle of the aneurism needle work down between the artery and the wind-pipe, and between the vein and artery, using care not to injure the vein. Now take the hook end of the aneurism needle and start in between the vein and the artery, pointing the hook towards the wind-pipe. Raise the artery gently and place the forceps under, (as per cut).

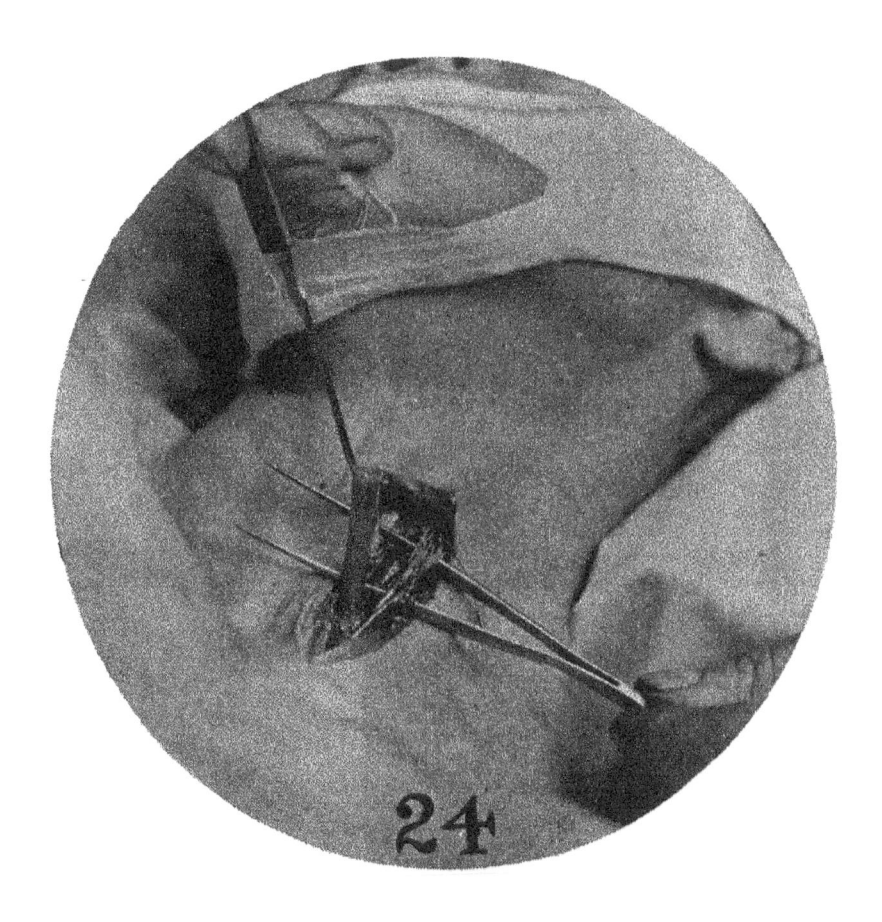

There is still another sheath covering the artery. Take the hook end of the aneurism needle, and scratch along on the top of the sheath to open it. Then lift the artery with the aneurism needle, let the sheath drop (as per cut) and place the forceps under the artery.

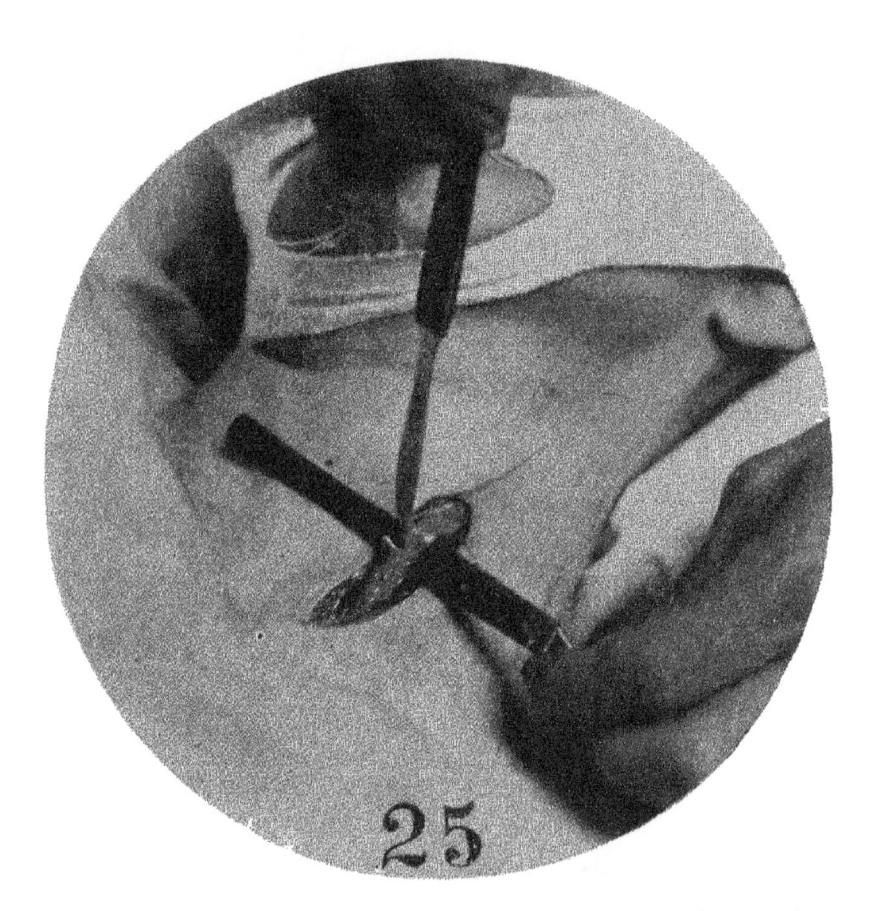

Now place the handle of the aneurism needle under the artery, and take the forceps out. Next take the scalpel and nick the artery (as per cut).

26

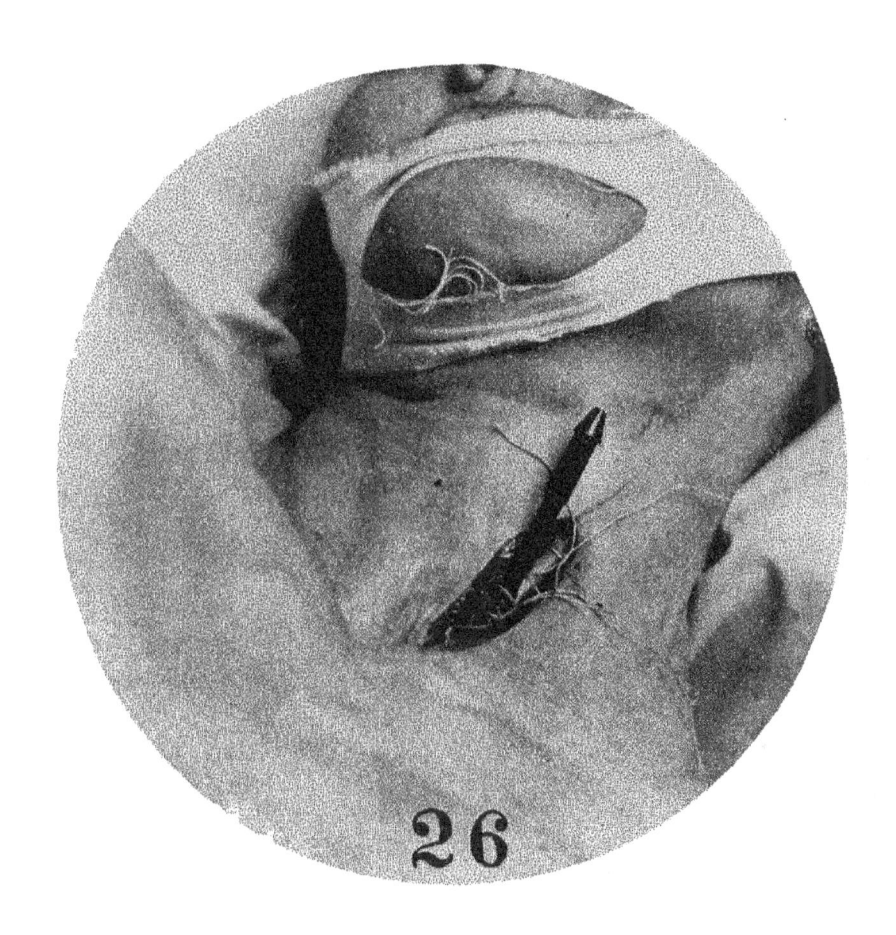

Take two pieces of waxed thread and put them under the artery, one at each end of the incision. Now take the arterial tube and place it in the artery, pointing toward the heart. Then tie one hard knot and one bow knot around the artery and tube, behind the shoulder of the tube. Tie the other thread loosely around the artery (as per cut), until the fluid makes its appearance while you are injecting the body. Then tie it tightly.

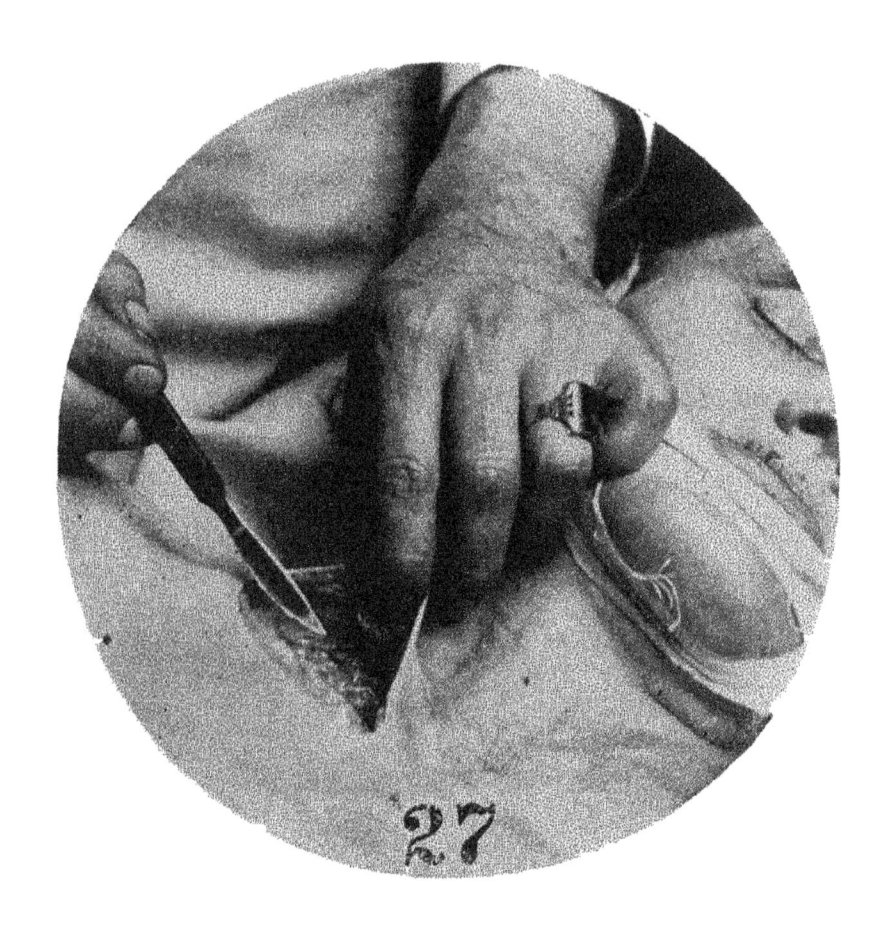

## TO RAISE THE COMMON CAROTID ARTERY.
### TRANSVERSE INCISION.

Take the scalpel and make an incision along the center of the cavicle or collar-bone, beginning in the center, and making the incision from two to two and a half inches long, cutting through to the bone. Then dissect the skin upward. Now cut off the muscle which is attached to the cavicle (as per cut). The muscle will now draw up and not interfere.

28

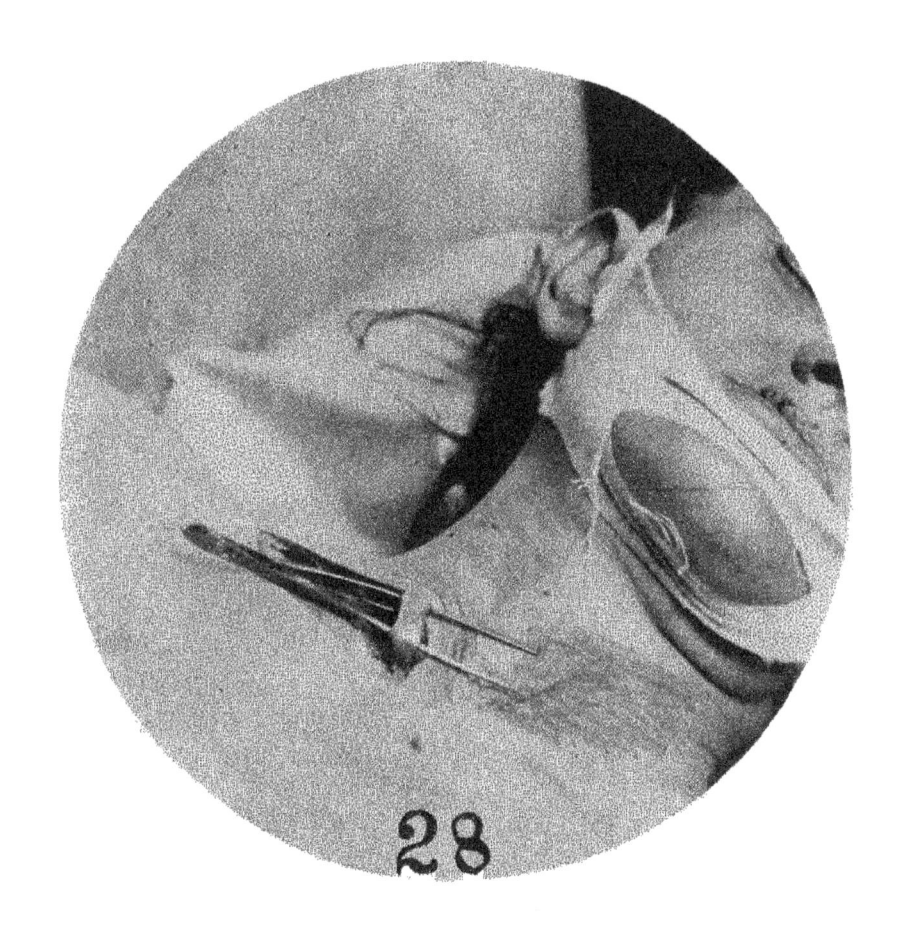

Take the hook end of the aneurism needle and tear the deep fascia which lies directly over the artery and vein. Then tear the sheath from off the artery which lies next the wind-pipe. With the handle end of the aneurism needle separate the artery from he wind-pipe and then from the vein, using care not to rupture the vein. Next pass the hook of the aneurism needle between the vein and the artery, pointing towards the wind-pipe. Raise the artery carefully and place the forceps under it (as per cut).

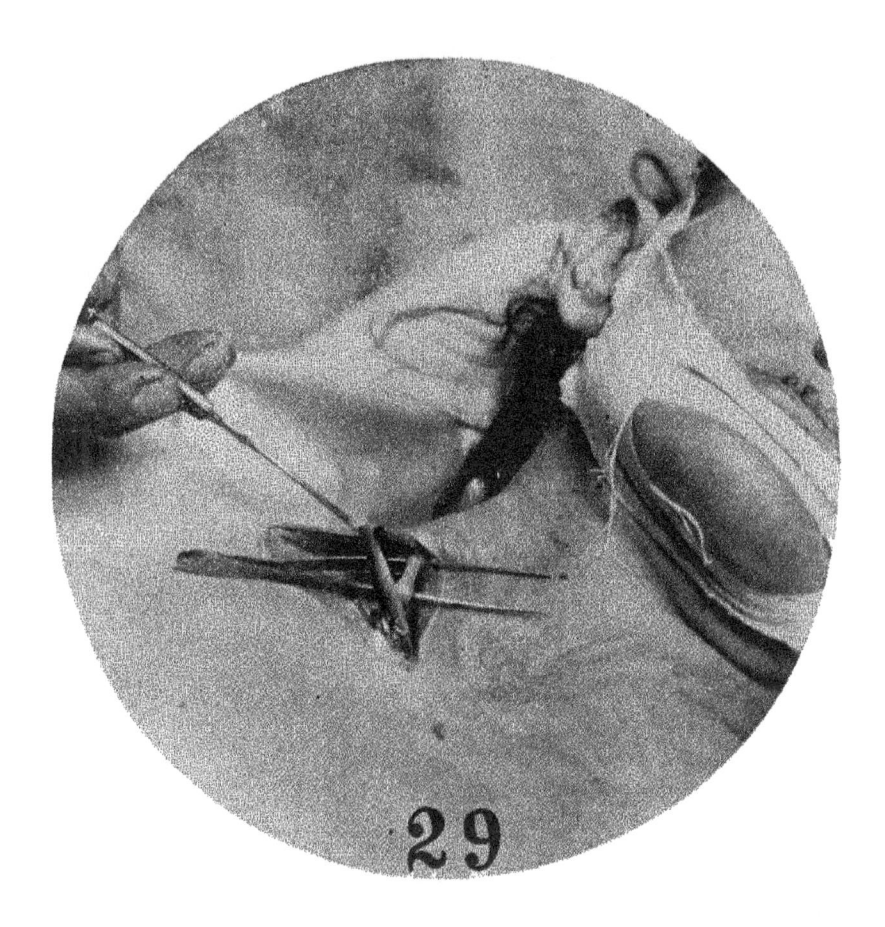

Take the hook end of the aneurism needle and scratch along the top of the sheath that surrounds the artery, to open it. Raise the artery, let the sheath drop (as per cut) and place the forceps under the artery.

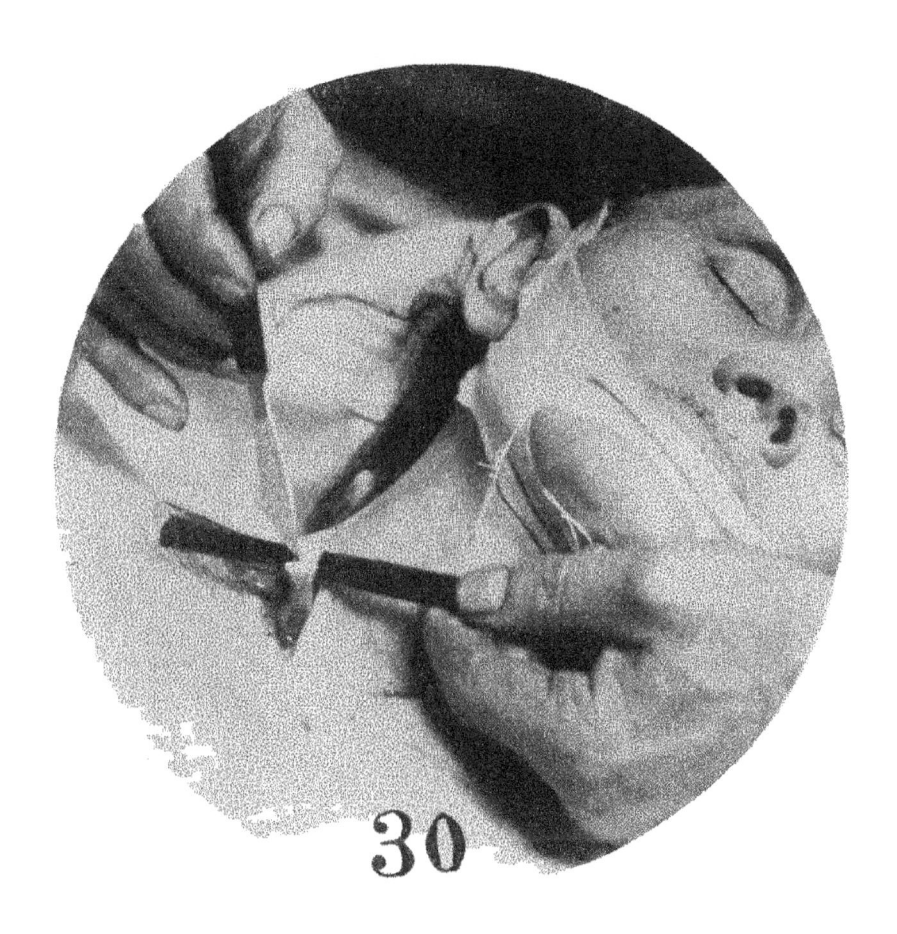

Take the handle end of the aneurism needle, put it under the artery and draw the forceps out. Then take the scalpel and make an incision (as per cut).

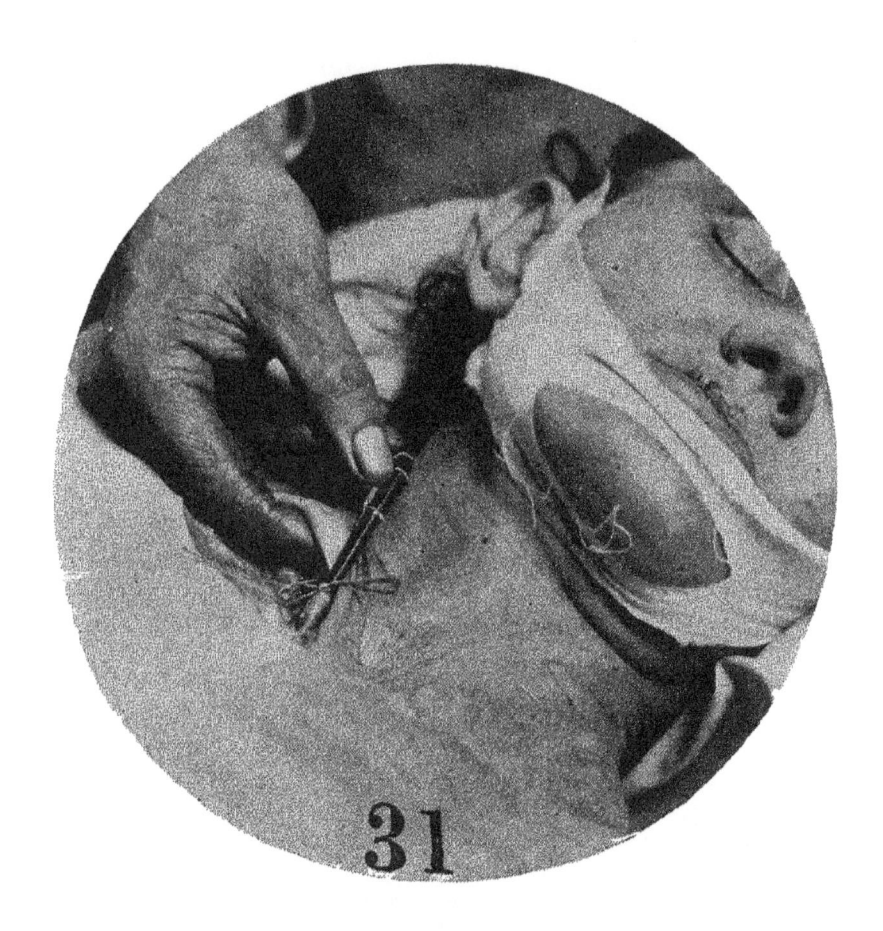

Place the arterial tube in the artery, pointing toward the heart. Then take a piece of waxed thread and tie one hard and one bow knot behind the shoulder of the arterial tube. Take another piece of waxed thread and tie it loosely around the artery above the tube (as per cut). Keep it tied loosely until the fluid makes its appearance, while you are injecting the body. Then tie it tightly.

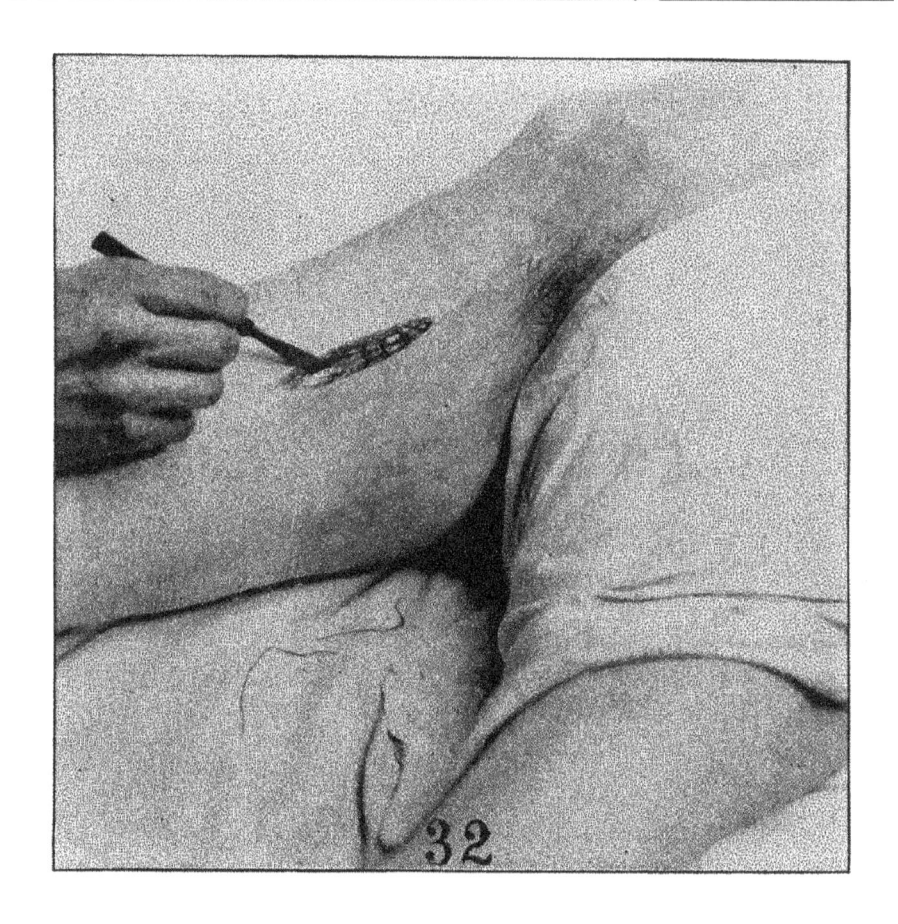

## TO LOCATE AND RAISE THE FEMORAL ARTERY.

Upon raising the knee a little you will notice three valleys running down the limb, commencing where the limb is attached to the trunk. With the fingers trace the middle valley down from one and a half to two inches, from where the limb joins the trunk. Then begin the incision from that point, cutting downward from about two to two and a half inches, and from one to two inches deep (as per cut). Underlying this will be found the layer of deep fascia, which may be split with the point of the scalpel (using great care not to cut the vein or artery). Underneath this deep fascia there is a layer of fatty substance from one-eighth to one quarter of an inch thick, overlying the artery.

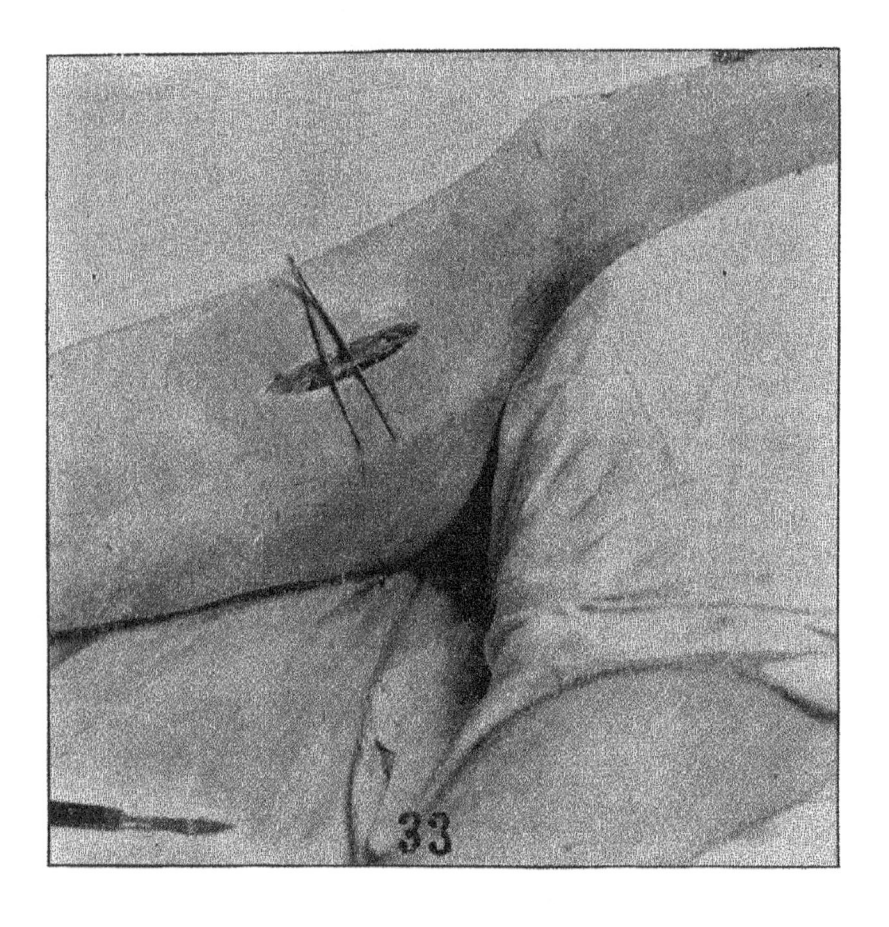

Take the handle end of the aneurism needle and work down to the artery. With the hook end of the needle open the sheath on top of the artery. Next take the handle end of the needle and work it down between the artery and vein on both sides. Then take the hook end of the needle, raise the artery and place the forceps under it (as per cut).

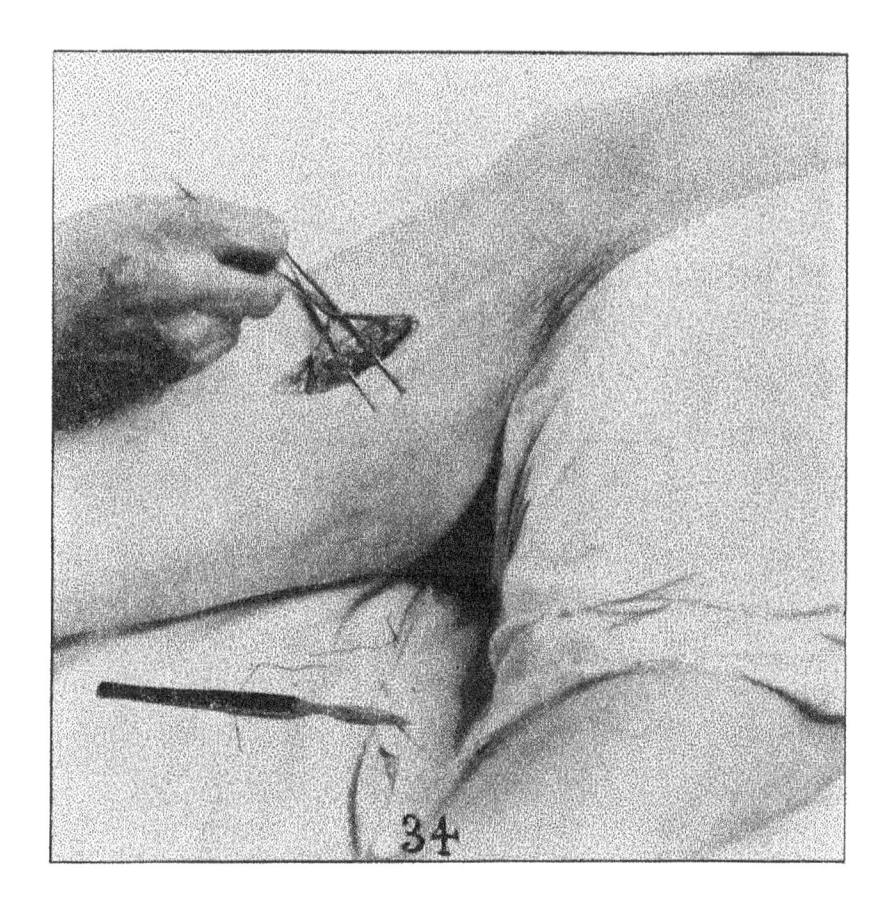

Take the hook end of the aneurism needle, open the sheath that covers the artery, and then raise the artery and let the sheath drop (as per cut). Then place the forceps under it.

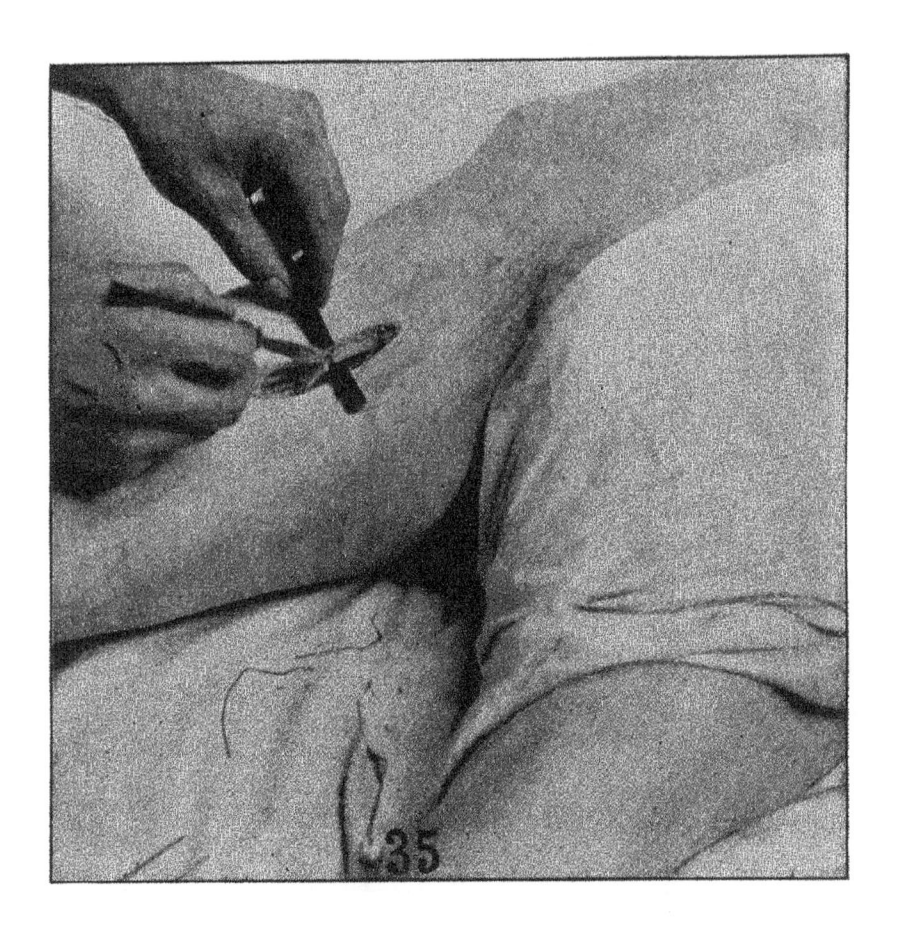

Take the aneurism needle, place it under the artery and take out the forceps. Then take the scalpel and make an incision (as per cut).

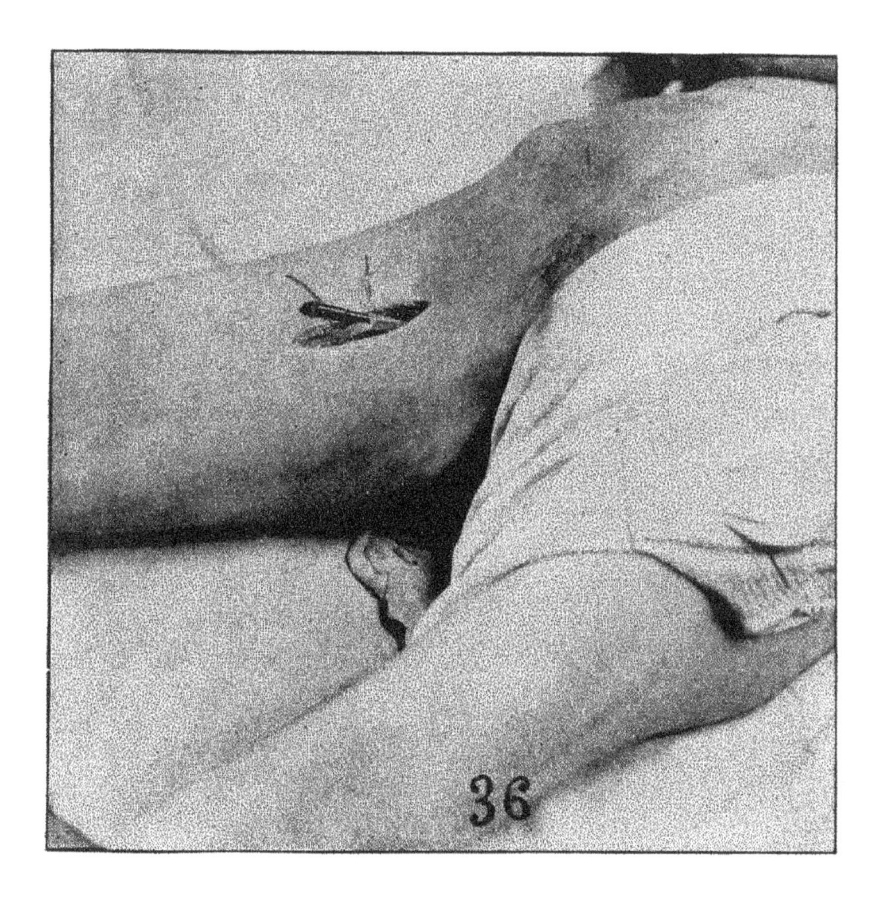

Take two pieces of waxed thread and put them under the artery, one at each end of the incision. Then place the arterial tube in the artery. Next tie one thread around the artery and tube in one hard and one bow knot, behind the shoulder of the tube. Tie the other thread in a loose knot around the artery (as per cut). When the fluid makes its appearance, while you are injecting the body, tie it tightly.

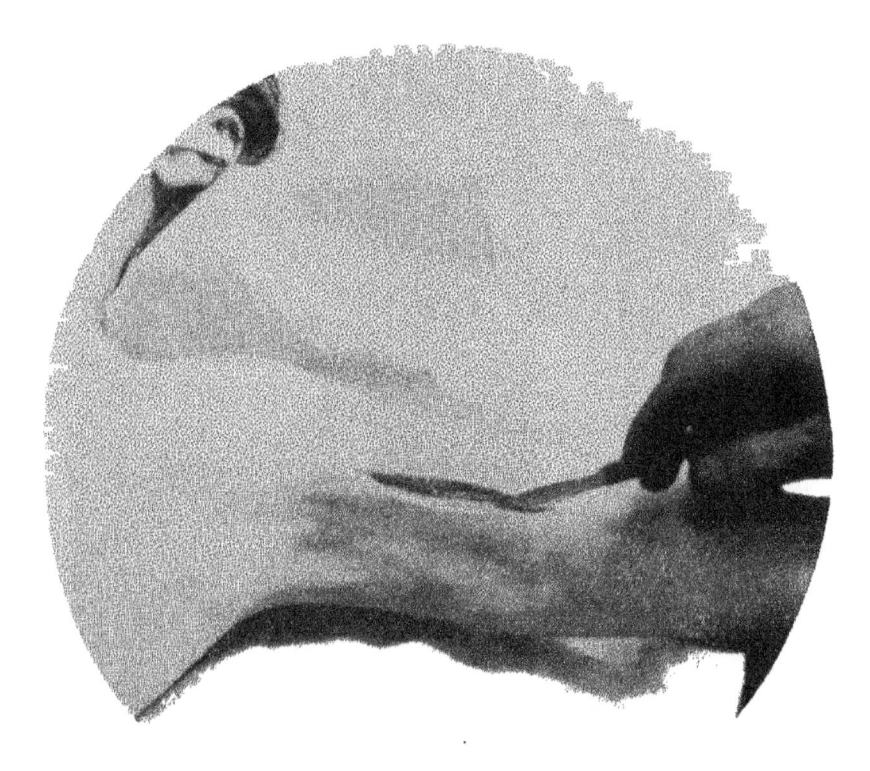

## 37

### TO LOCATE AND RAISE THE BASILIC VEIN.

First trace the inner and under border of the biceps muscle of the left arm in the middle and upper third of the arm. Find the medium nerve, to the inner side of which you will find the basilic vein. Then take the scalpel and make an incision, just through the skin, from one and one-half to two and a half inches long (as per cut).

38

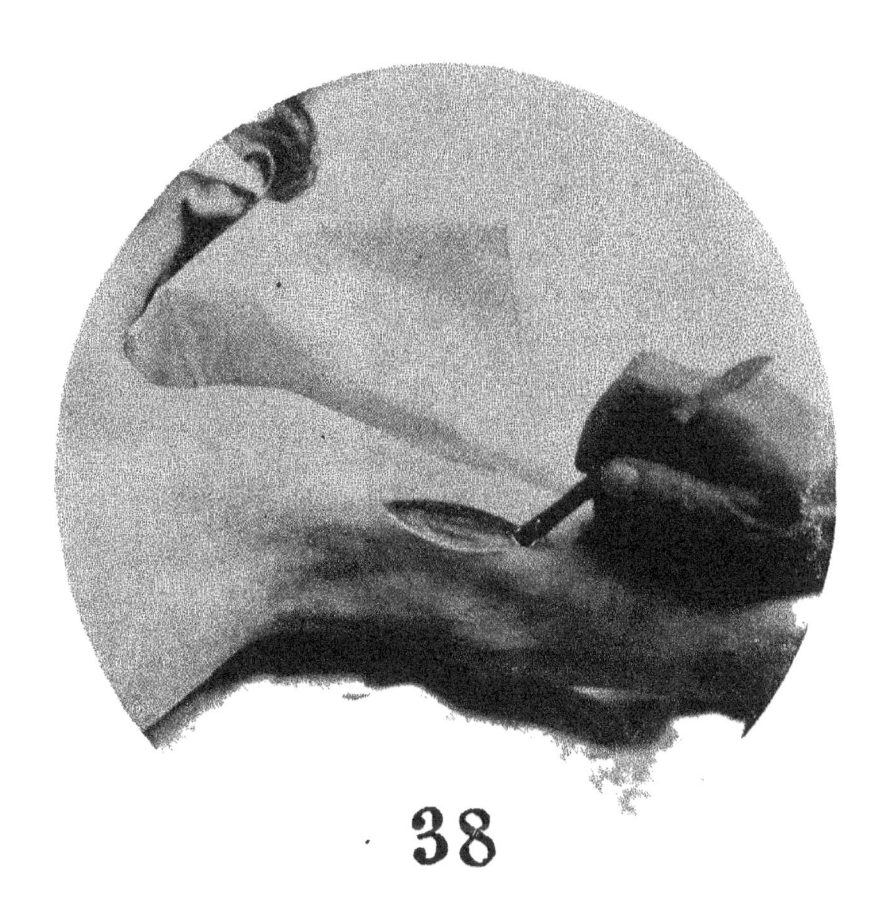

Take the handle end of the scalpel or aneurism needle and work down through the fatty substance to the deep fascia (as per cut).

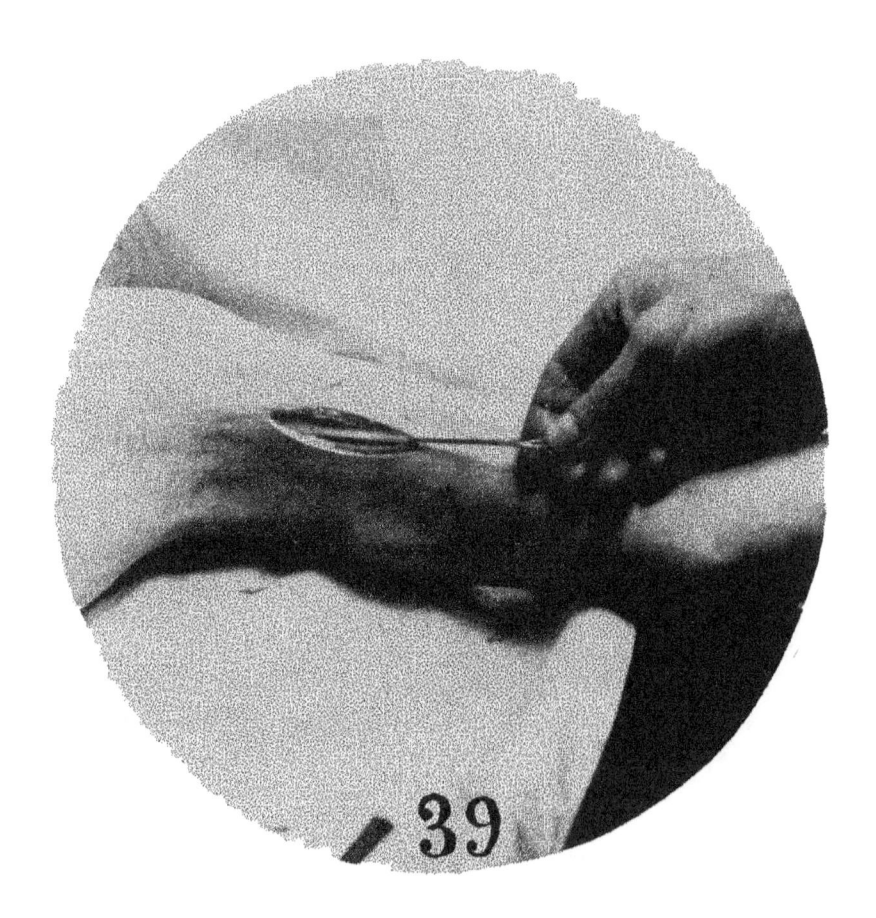

Take the sharp end of the fascia needle and puncture the deep fascia at the lower end of the incision. Next reverse the fascia needle, enter the puncture and run up under the deep fascia with the groove of the needle up (as per cut).

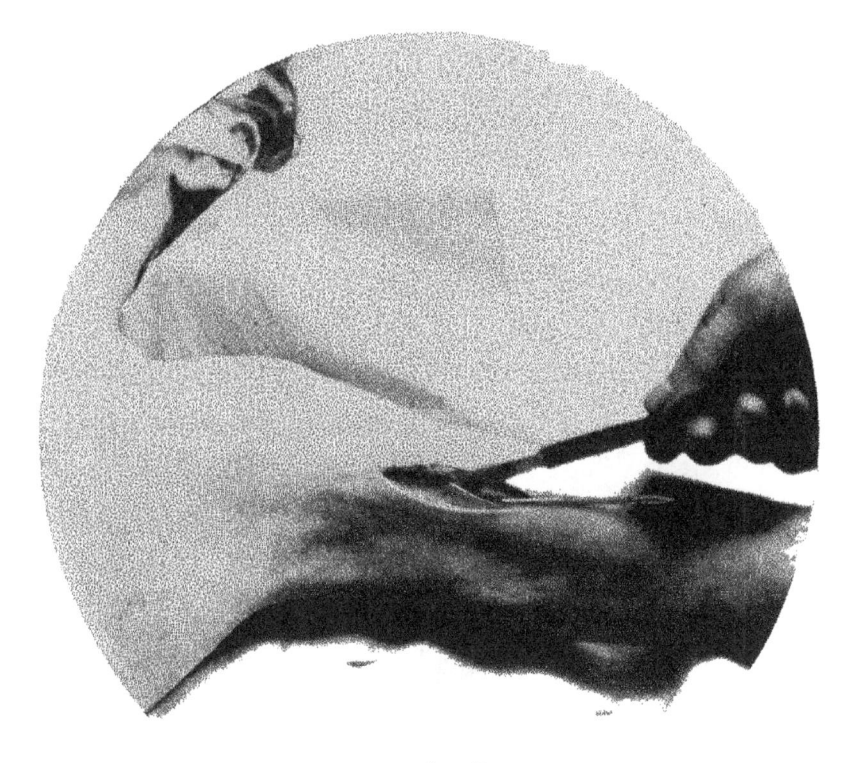

## 40

Take the scalpel and lay its back in the groove of the fascia needle; then rip the deep fascia the length of the incision (as per cut).

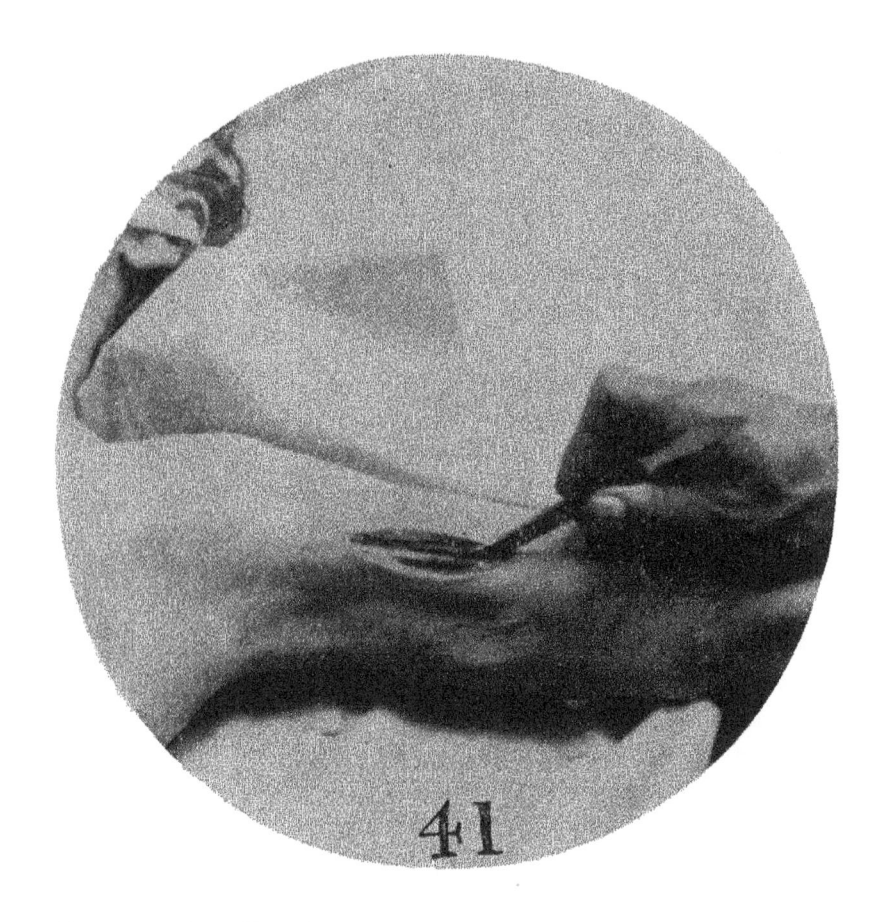

Take the handle of the aneurism needle or scalpel and work down through the fatty substance to the vein. Then work on down between the vein and nerve on the outer side of the vein, and between the vein and muscle on the inner side (as per cut).

42

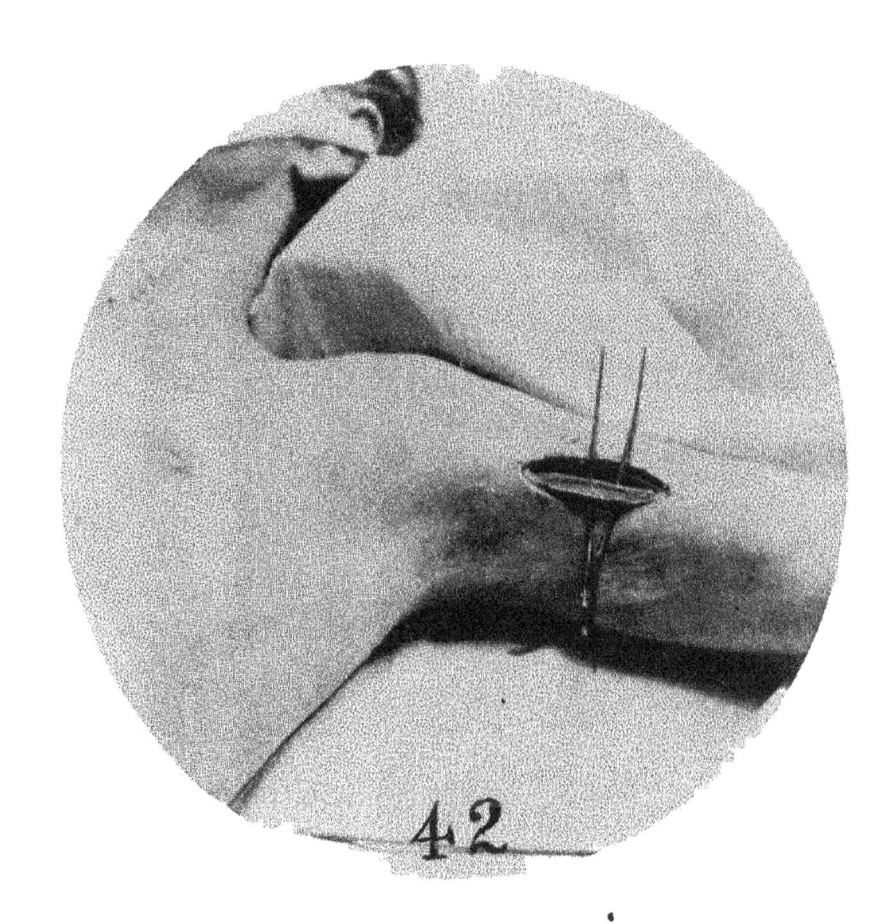

Then take the aneurism needle, raise the vein and put the forceps under it (as per cut).

43

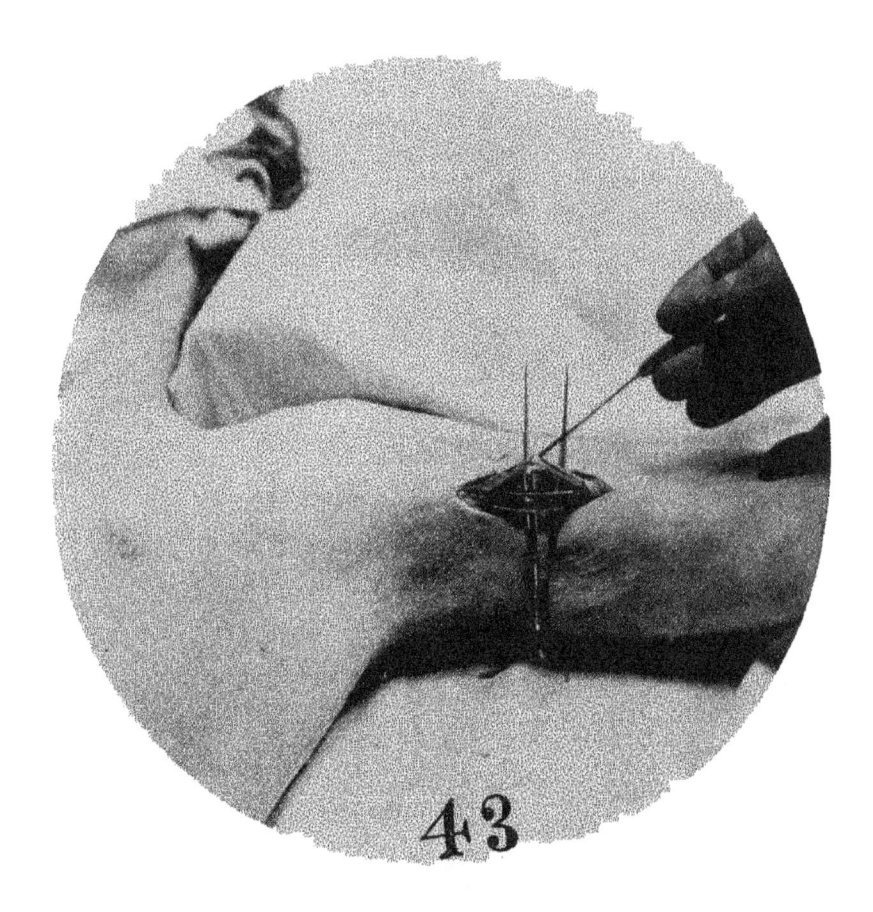

Take the hook end of the aneurism needle and scratch on the top of the sheath that surrounds the vein to open it. Now take the aneurism needle, raise the vein, let the sheath drop (as per cut) and put the forceps under the vein.

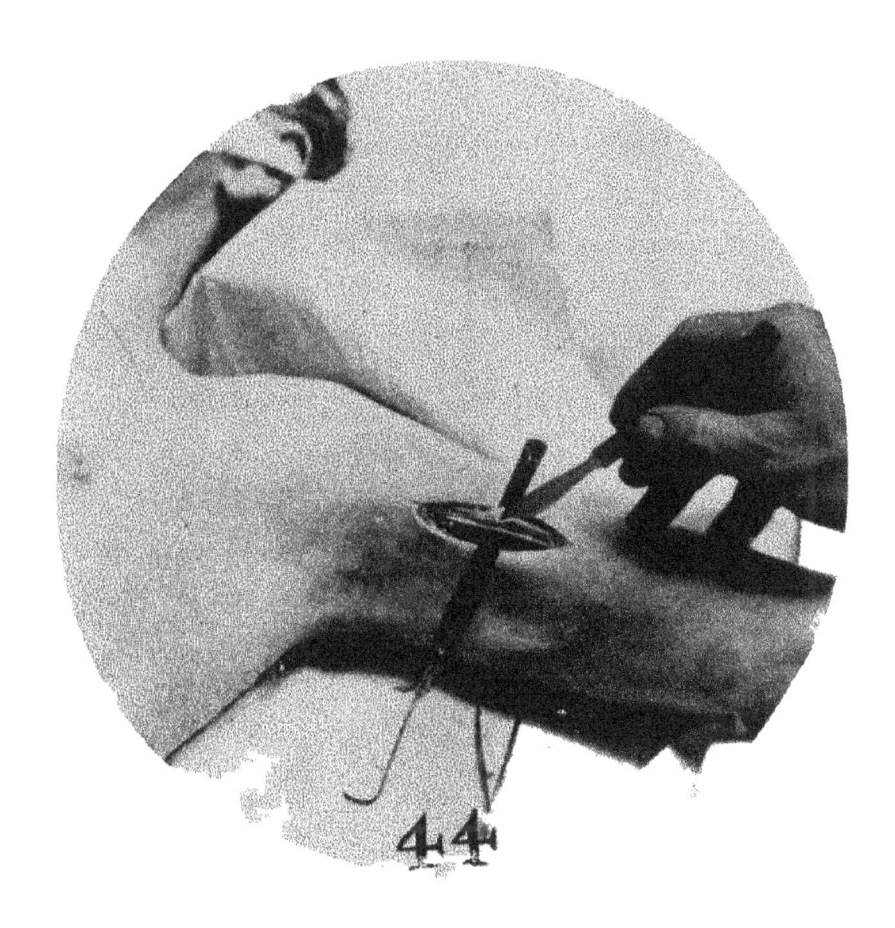

Take the aneurism needle, place it under the vein and take the forceps out. Then take the scalpel and nick the vein (as per cut).

52 ESPY'S EMBALMER.

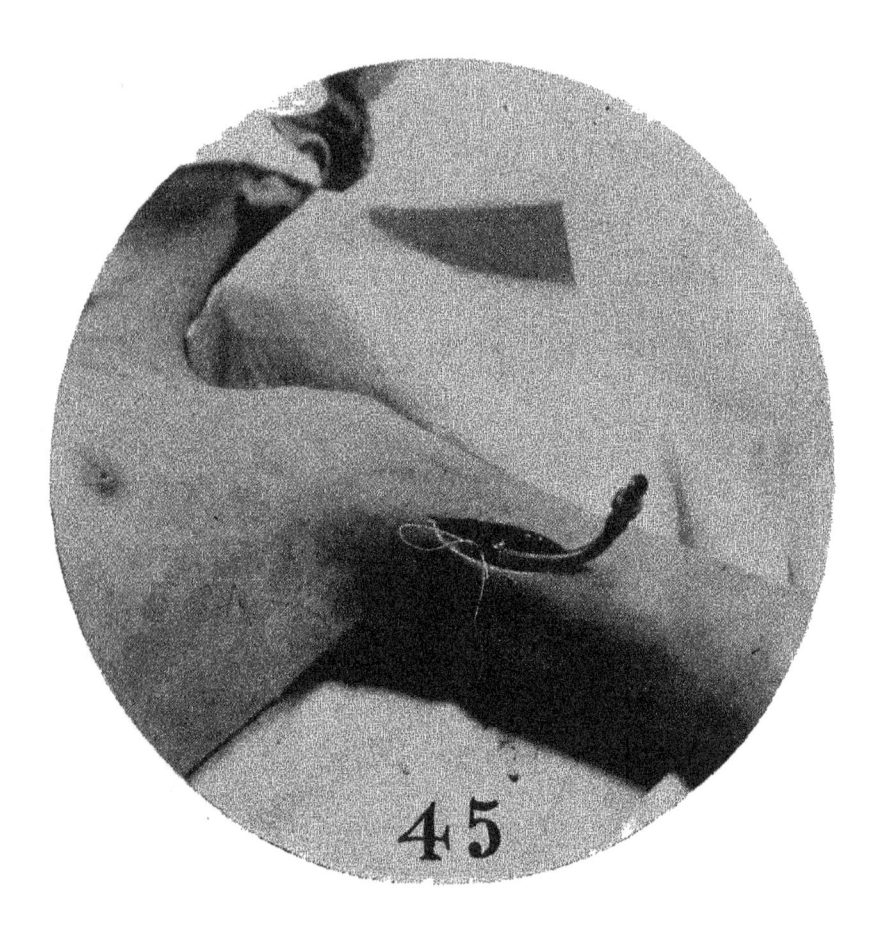

45

Take two pieces of waxed thread and place them under the vein, one at each end of the incision. Then take the basilic vein tube and cover it with vaseline. Enter the vein and follow it up until you enter the right auricle of the heart. Then tie one hard knot and one bow knot around the vein and tube. Tie the other thread loosely around the vein (as per cut). When through drawing blood, withdraw the tube and tie both threads, tightly.

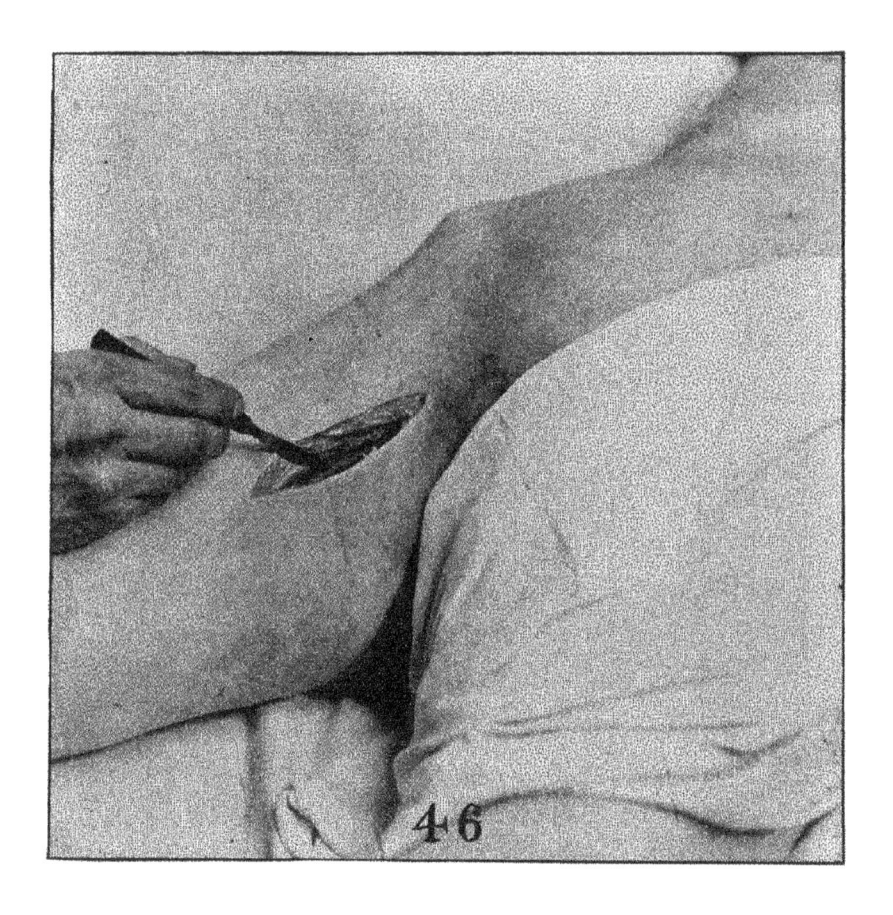

## TO LOCATE AND RAISE THE FEMORAL VEIN.

For this ALWAYS use the RIGHT leg. Upon raising the knee ightly you will find three valleys; underlying the middle one and at the point where the leg joins the trunk, lie the femoral vein and artery, the vein being on the inner side.

Take the scalpel and make an incision, commencing where the leg is attached to the trunk, and cutting downward. Follow this valley for about two to two and a half inches, and cut in carefully to the deep fascia (as per cut).

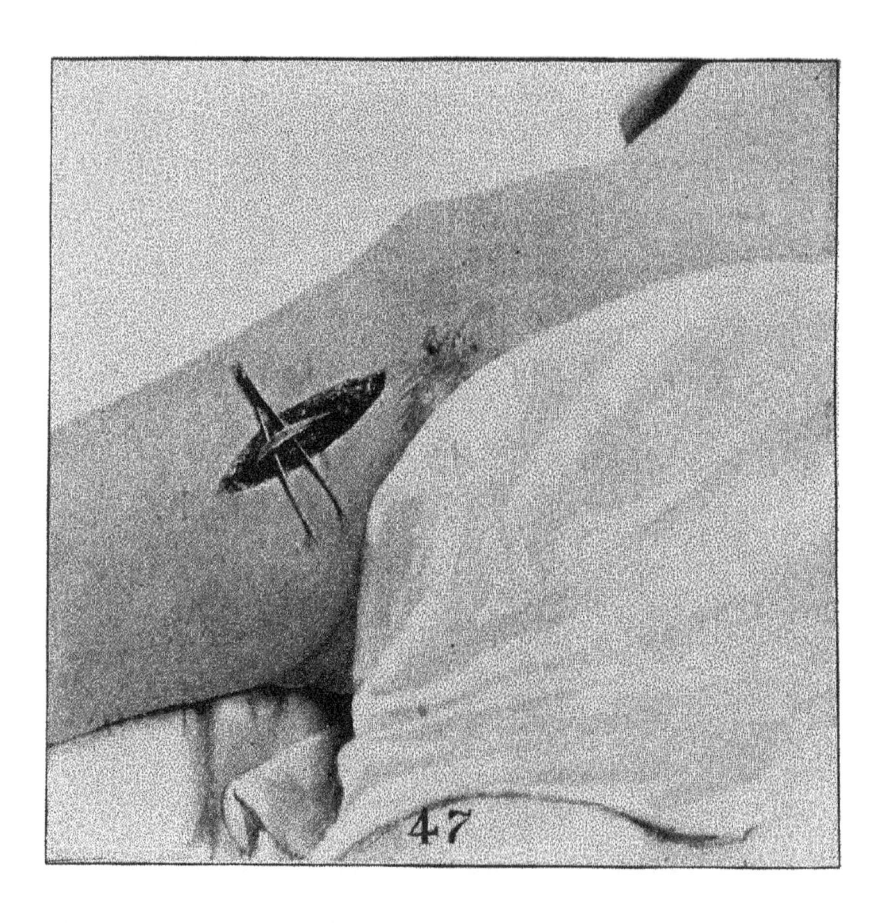

Take the handle end of the aneurism needle and split the deep fascia, being careful not to injure any of the branches of the artery or vein. Next separate the vein from the artery on the one side, and the vein from the muscle on the other. Take the hook end of the aneurism needle, raise the vein and place the forceps under it (as per cut).

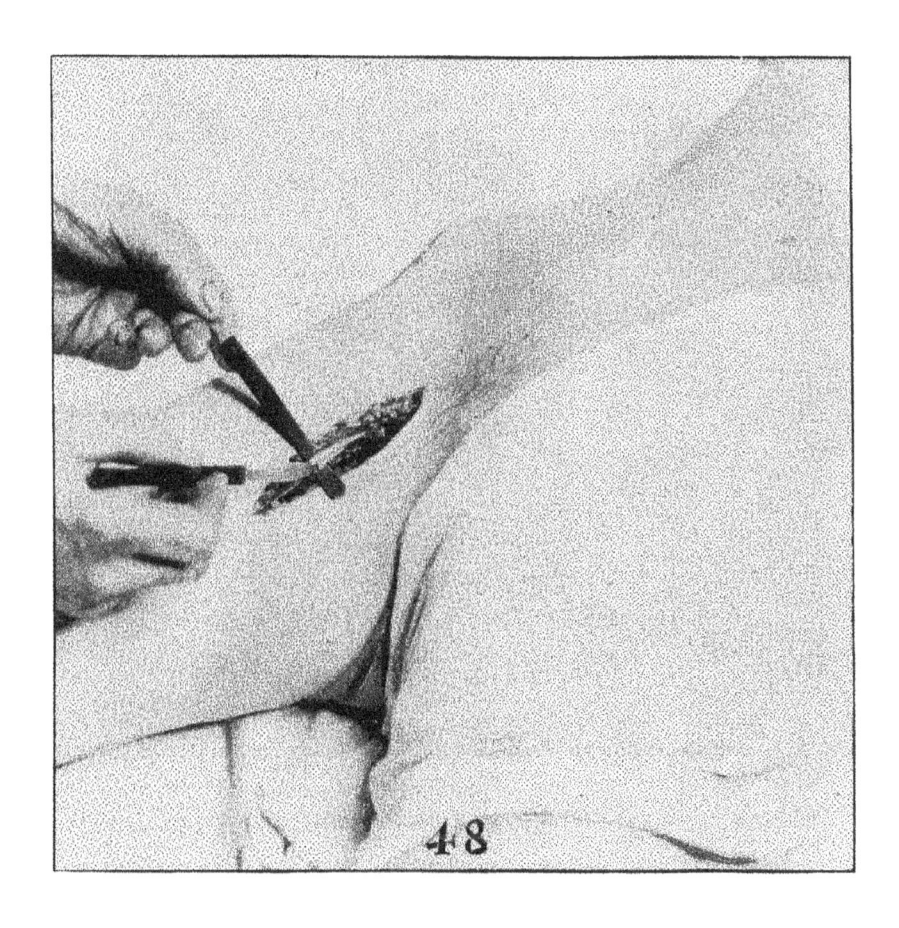

Take the handle end of the aneurism needle and place it under the vein and draw out the forceps. Then take the scalpel and make an incision in the vein (as per cut).

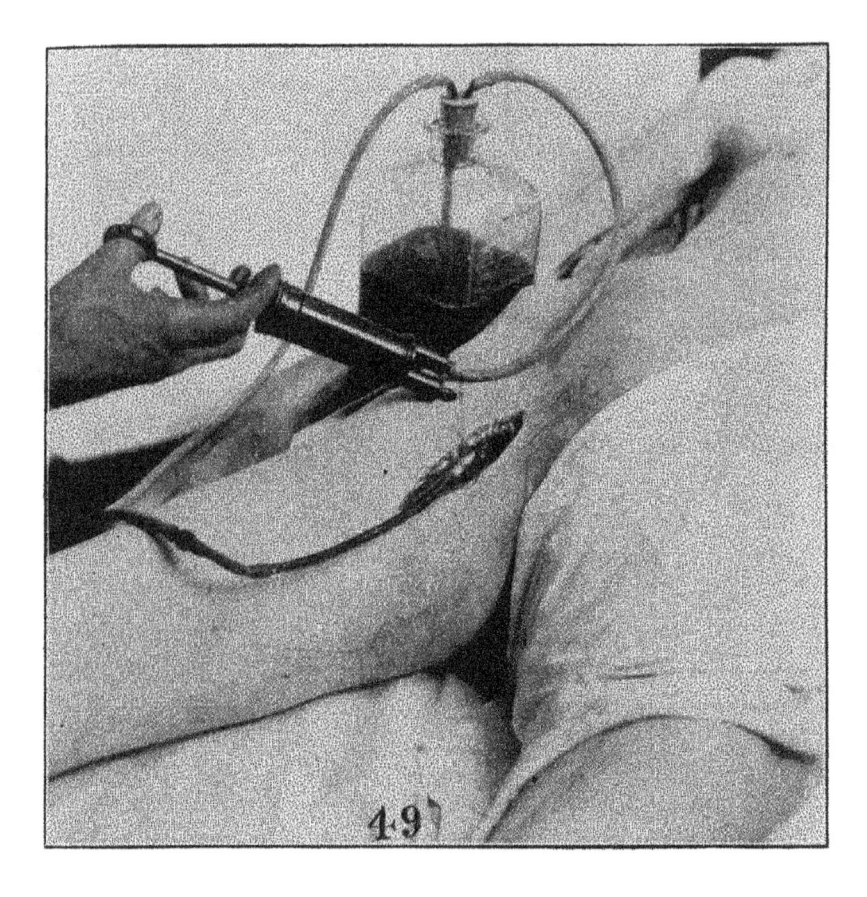

Take two pieces of waxed thread, and put them under the vein, one at each end of the incision. Now take the femoral vein tube, cover it with vaseline, and attach it to the aspirator; (the aspirator being in an empty bottle). Then enter the vein with the tube and follow it up into the right auricle. Tie one thread in one hard and one bow knot around the vein and tube. Tie the other thread tightly around the vein (as per cut). When through drawing blood, withdraw the tube and tie the first thread tightly.

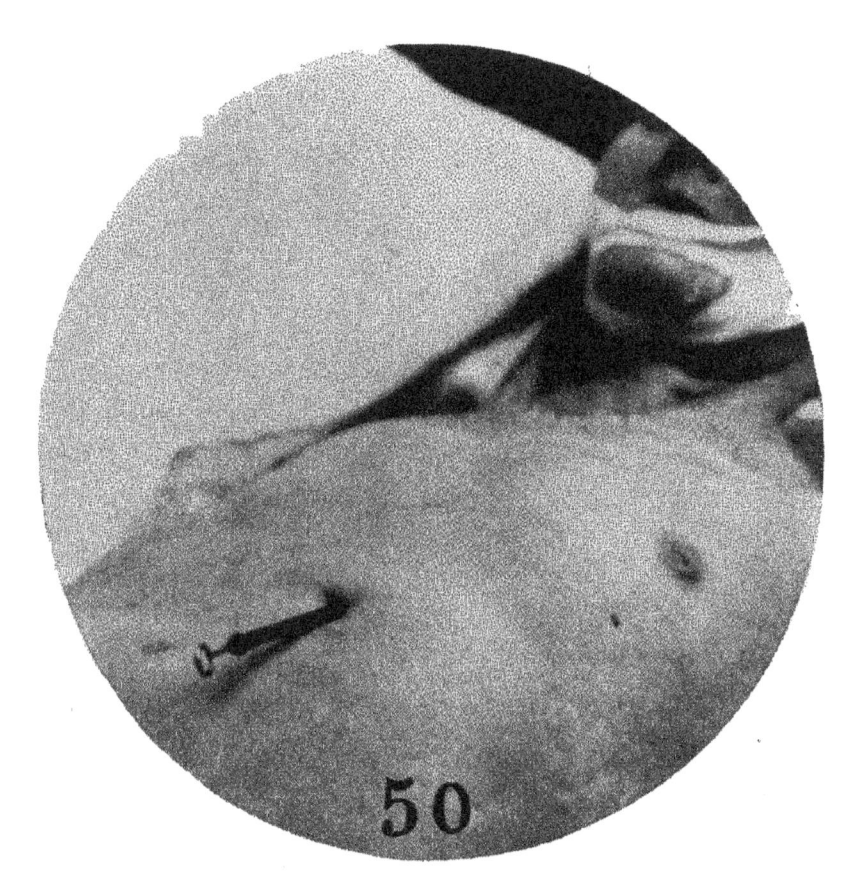

## TAPPING THE RIGHT VENTRICLE OF THE HEART.

Take a twelve-inch trocar and enter the abdominal cavity, two inches below the breast bone and one inch to the left, going straight in. Then point it upward and go toward the lobe of the right ear. Then puncture the diaphram and go on up and puncture the pericardium or heart sac. Now push in the rod to protect the point until you strike the heart, and after you have fairly gotten on to the heart, pull the rod out a short distance, keeping the trocar pointed toward the lobe of the right ear. Now push the trocar into the heart a distance of from one to one and a half inches (as per cut No. 50). Then push the rod in, turn it around and draw it out. If there is blood on the end of it, you are all right; but if not, draw the trocar out of the heart and push the rod in again to protect the point, and feel around until you get fairly onto the heart, then pull out the rod a short distance and push in the trocar an inch and a half. Push in the rod, turn it around and draw it out. If no blood appears keep this up until you succeed.

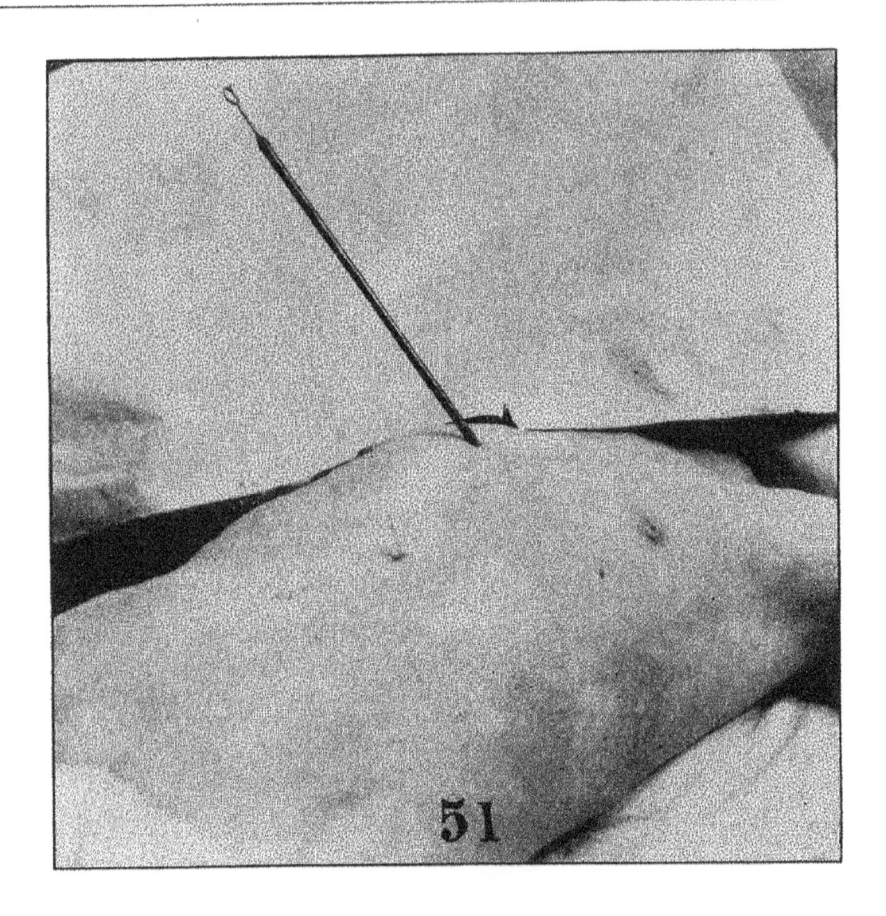

## TAPPING THE RIGHT AURICLE OF THE HEART.

Count the ribs downward, beginning at the first rib (always on the right side), but do not count the cavicle or collar-bone. The first rib is a very short one and lies almost directly beneath the cavicle or collar-bone. Count to the space between the third and fourth ribs, about one-half inch to the right of the sternum or breast-bone.

Take the trocar and point it downward and to the left. After going through the chest wall, push the rod in to protect the point. Feel around until you have struck the heart, which will be some three or four inches on a line to the left and downward. Then pull out the rod and push the trocar into the heart from one to one and a quarter inches. Now push the rod in, turn it around and pull it out; if there is no blood on it, push the trocar in a little farther until you succeed in getting blood (as per cut No. 51).

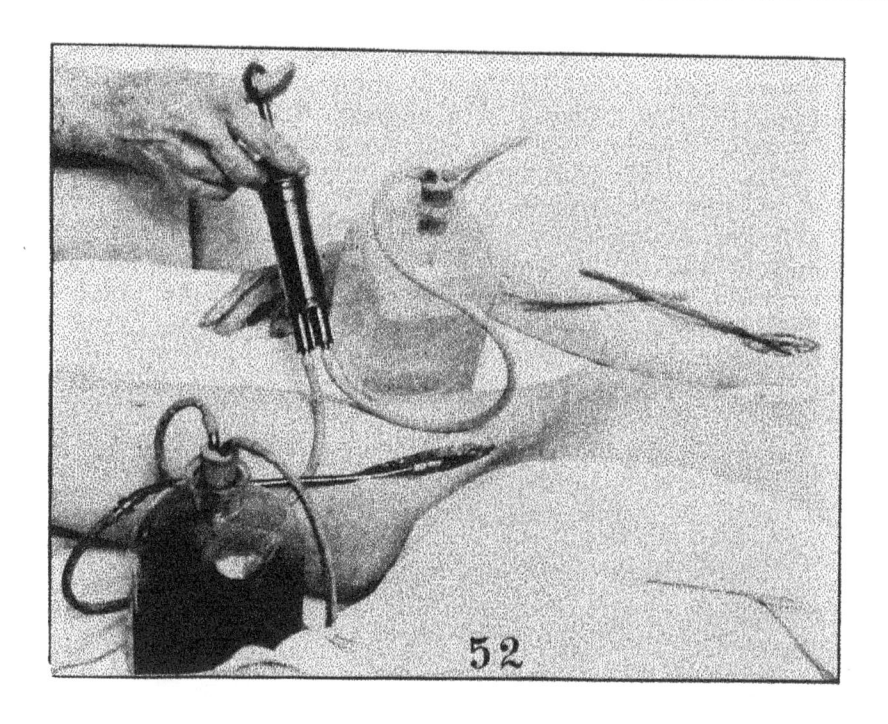

## DRAWING BLOOD FROM THE HEART AND DRAINING THE BODY.

It is not always necessary to drain the body of blood, but when it is, it is VERY necessary, for there is no matter about the body that gives us as much trouble as the blood. There are four ways to do this. The one most preferable is by using the femoral vein. Lift it according to instructions and accompanying cuts, Nos. 46 to 50. Attach the drawing side of the pump to the aspirator. Always use the pump, for there is no bulb made strong enough to draw the blood, for when you are drawing it you are causing a vacuum. Sometimes you can get but very little blood on that account. Now, there is a way to overcome that difficulty, and that is to take another aspirator or injector and attach to one of the four arteries given, viz.: the radial, brachial, carotid or femoral. The two best are the radial and brachial arteries. Attach the aspirator or injector to the arterial tube in the artery which you use; place the injector in a bottle full of fluid and attach the injecting side of the pump to the aspirator or injector. Then inject and aspirate at the same stroke of the pump (as per cut No. 52). This will inject into the arteries and through the capillaries into the veins, back of the blood, and will push the blood ahead of the fluid and fill the vacuum you are causing; or you can aspirate for a while, then inject, and alternately. You will have the best results by keeping this up, until the fluid appears through the femoral vein tube. When it appears, you will have nearly all the blood drawn. When you inject, you may use a bulb injector or a syringe. For ordinary injecting the bulb injector is as good as any; or you may draw the blood by using the basilic vein, the right ventricle, or the right auricle, in the same way as we use the femoral vein. It is always well to rub the head and face downward while drawing blood. Sometimes it is necessary to use cloths and hot water about the face and neck. If there is much coagulated blood, this will help very much. If the blood is coagulated so that you cannot draw any, inject a little hot salt water, which will dissolve the clots. Then aspirate and inject more salt water, and alternately until you have gotten a good flow of blood.

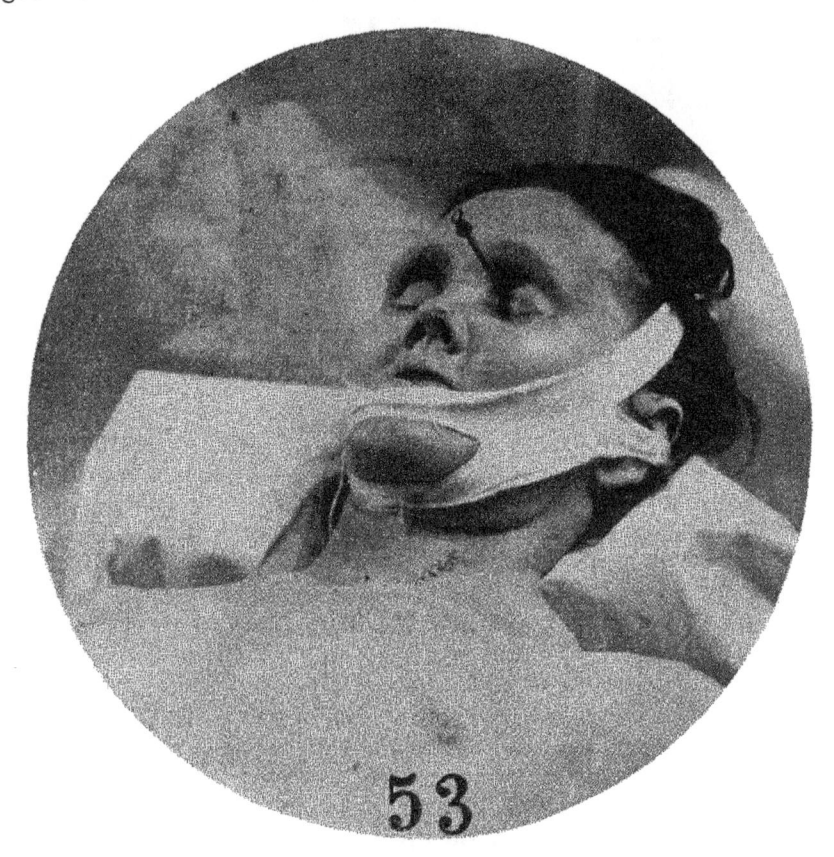

53

## TO INJECT THE BRAIN CAVITY.

In some cases this method may be used: To inject the brain cavity, first draw the blood, by entering with the small trocar the inner center of the eye and work on back, pointing downward, until you strike the back of the skull and rupture the Winepress (as per cut). Then attach the aspirator to the trocar and draw the blood. Now inject from one to three gills of fluid.

Use this method for alcoholism, paralysis, sunstroke, softening of the brain and like diseases.

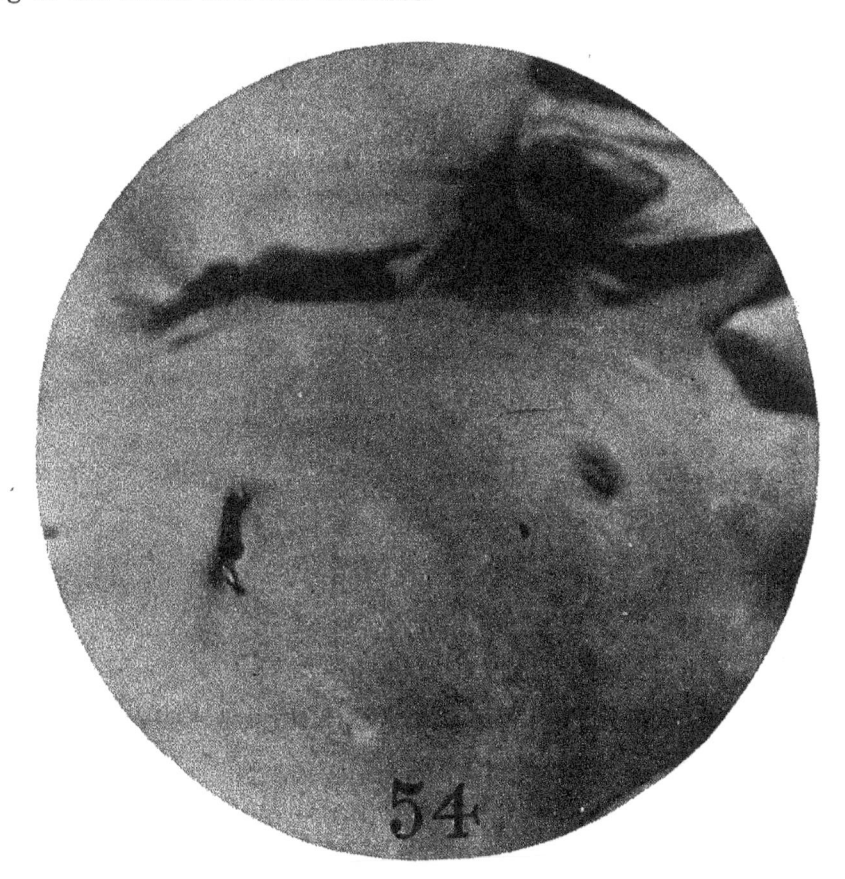

## TO INJECT THE THORACIO OR LUNG CAVITIES.
### BY ONE INCISION.

Take a twelve-inch trocar and enter the abdominal cavity, half way between the breast-bone and navel, and one inch to the left, going straight in and JUST through into the abdominal cavity. If there should be any gases, allow them to pass off, per instructions in another place. Then point the trocar toward the right shoulder and puncture the diaphram close up to the ribs. Next push it close up under the ribs (as per cut), using care not to rupture the lungs. Then inject Espy's Embalming Fluid. Draw the trocar back to the abdominal cavity and then point it toward the left shoulder and proceed as on the right side. Then inject the fluid.

**55**

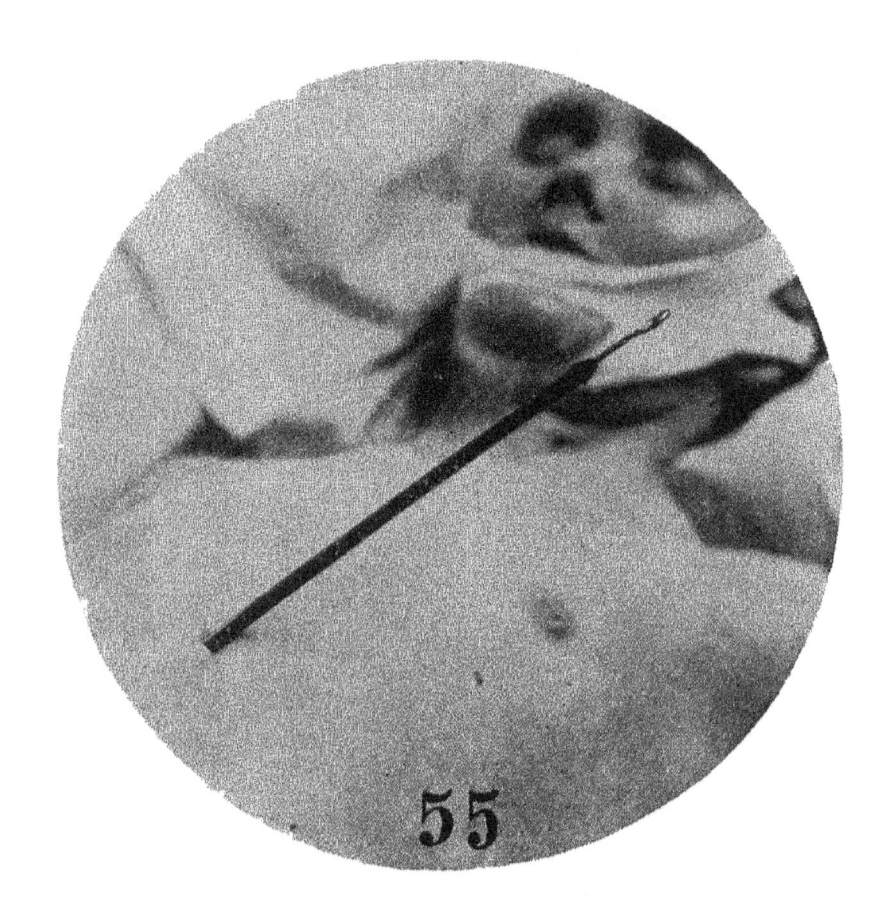

**TO INJECT THE ABDOMINAL CAVITY THROUGH THE SAME INCISION.**
**(AS CUT No. 54.)**

After you have injected the fluid, draw the trocar back into the abdominal cavity; point it downward (as per cut) and inject the fluid into each side of the abdominal cavity.

If you wish to puncture the stomach through this incision, point the trocar toward the left and downward. If there are any gases, allow them to escape per instructions in another place. Then inject the fluid.

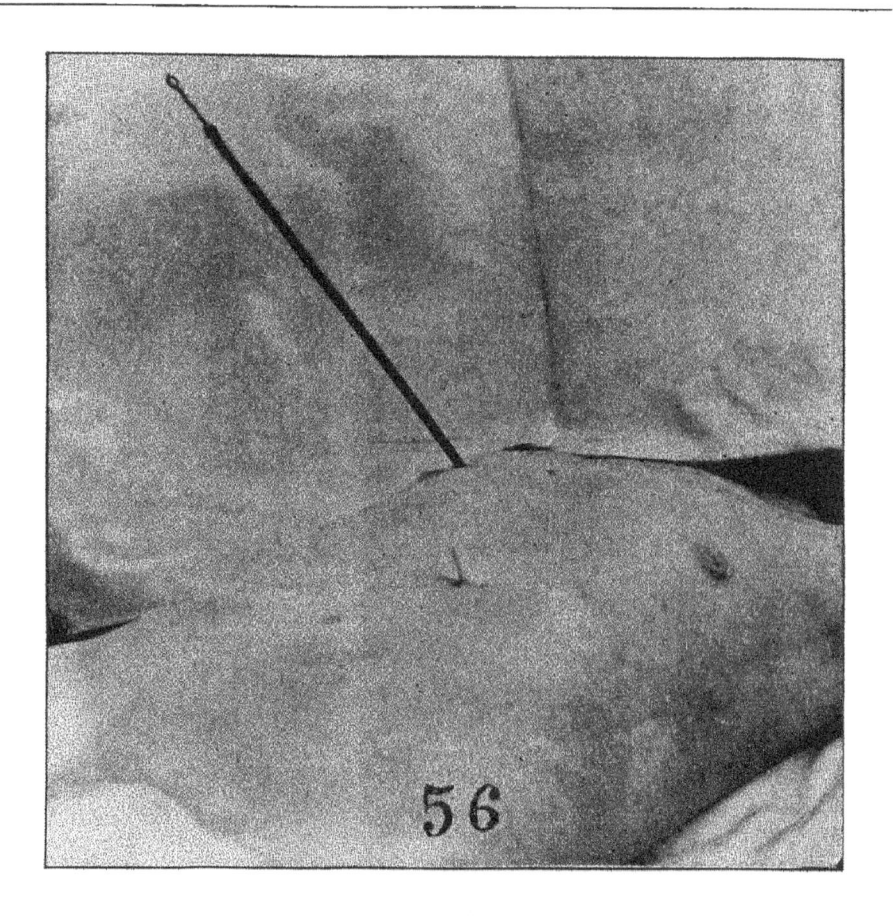

## TO INJECT THE THORACIC OR LUNG CAVITIES.

Count the ribs downward on the right side, commencing at the clavicle or collar bone, but do not count the clavicle or collar bone. Count down to the space between the fourth and fifth ribs, and down to the outer side of the nipple. (The first rib is a very short one and almost directly under the collar bone or clavicle.)

Take the trocar and enter the cavity at the space between the fourth and fifth ribs and to the outer side of the nipple. Go JUST THROUGH into the cavity (as per cut), using care not to rupture the lungs. If there are any gases, allow them to escape, per instructions in another place.

For the other side, count downward and proceed as on the right side.

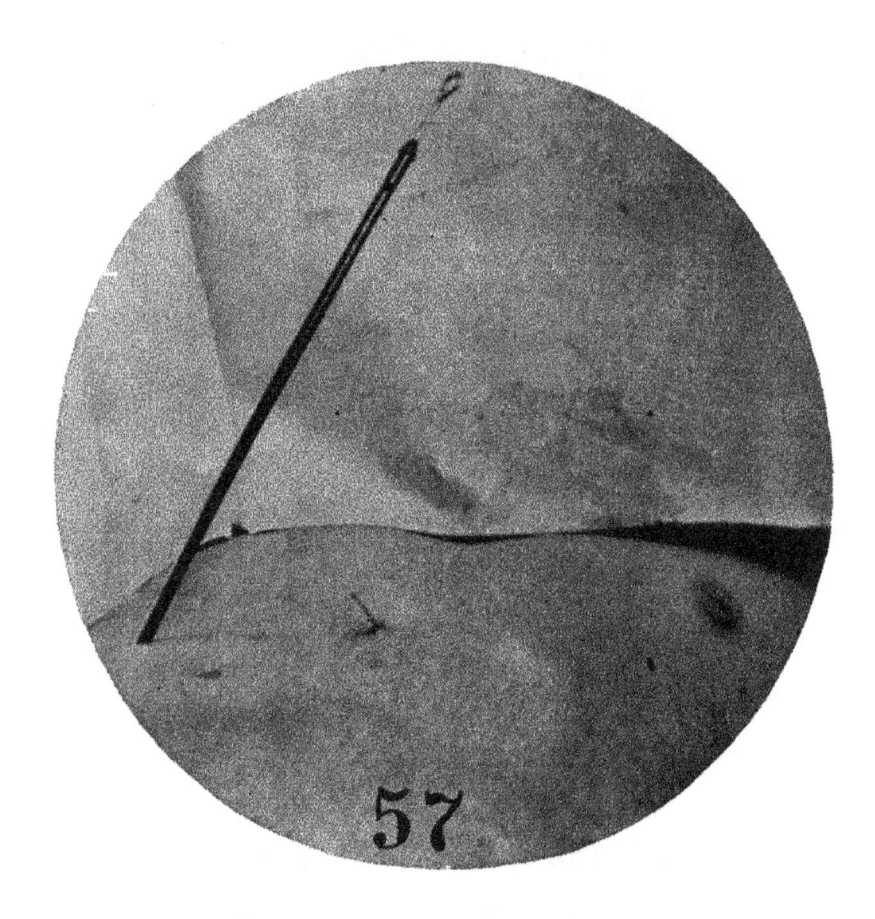

## TO INJECT THE ABDOMINAL CAVITY.

Take the trocar and make an incision just to one side of the navel (as per cut). If there are any gases, allow them to pass off per instructions in another place.

It is best to make three incisions for this reason. When all three cavities are injected through one incision, the diaphragm is punctured and the fluid that is injected into the thoracic or lung cavities will flow down into the abdominal cavity (for the body ought always be at an incline).

58

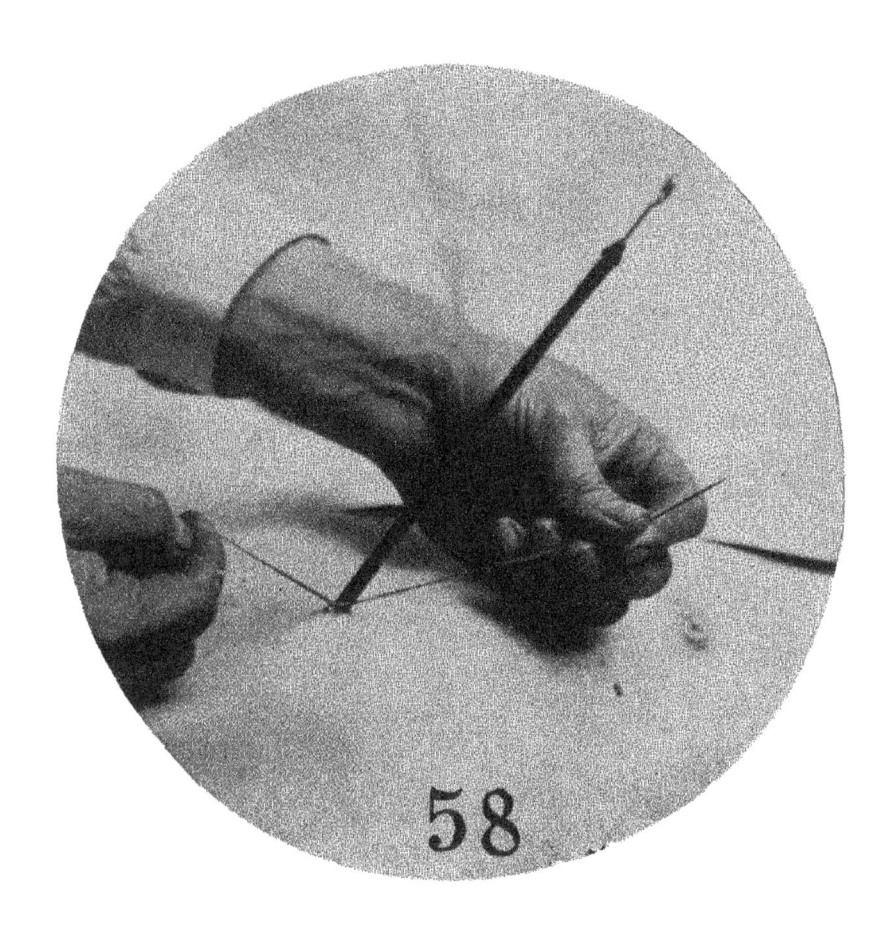

## TO SEW UP THE TROCAR INCISION.

Take a surgeon's needle and a piece of waxed thread and take a few stitches around the trocar, forming a draw-string. Draw it around the trocar and tie one knot (as per cut). Then draw out the trocar, draw the thread tightly and tie it.

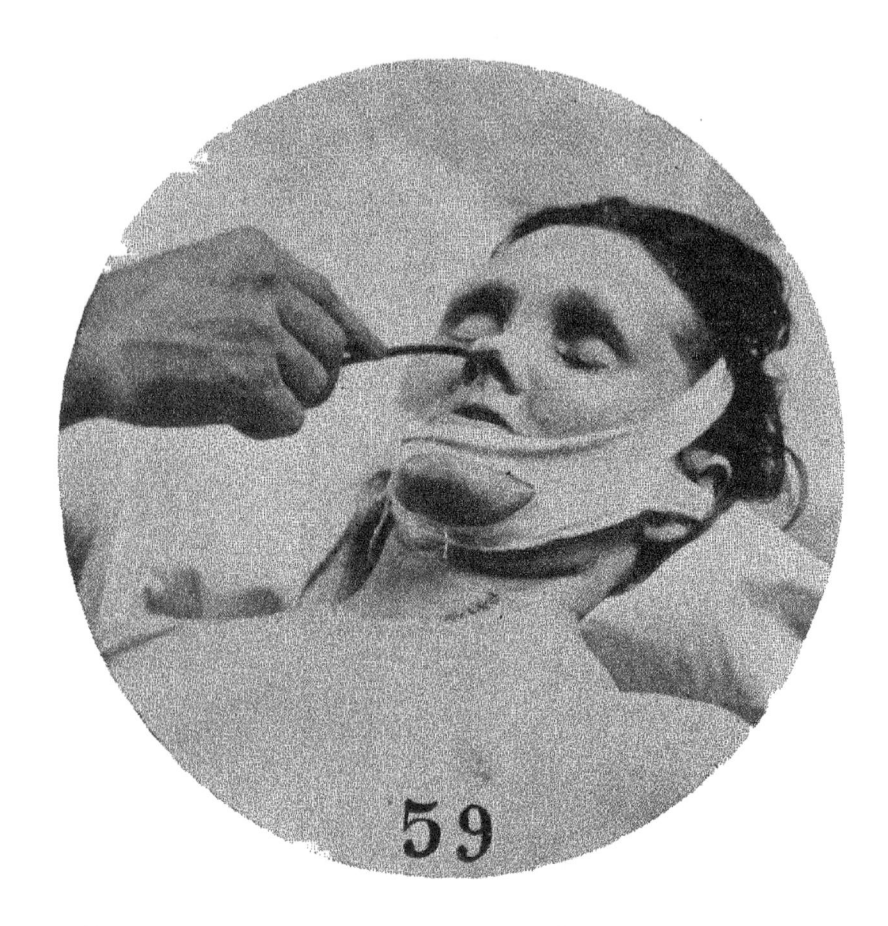

## TO INJECT THE STOMACH THROUGH THE NASAL PASSAGE.

Take the nasal tube and if it has not the proper curvature warm it in hot water, or by a lighted match, gas jet or lamp. Then lay it on a flat surface and bend it to the proper curvature. After it has cooled pass it down through the nostril, and, to allow the fluid to pass down into the stomach, raise the chin to enlarge the aperture of the æsophagus or gullet and work the nasal tube down into the æsophagus (as per cut). Then inject from one-half to one pint of Espy's Embalming Fluid.

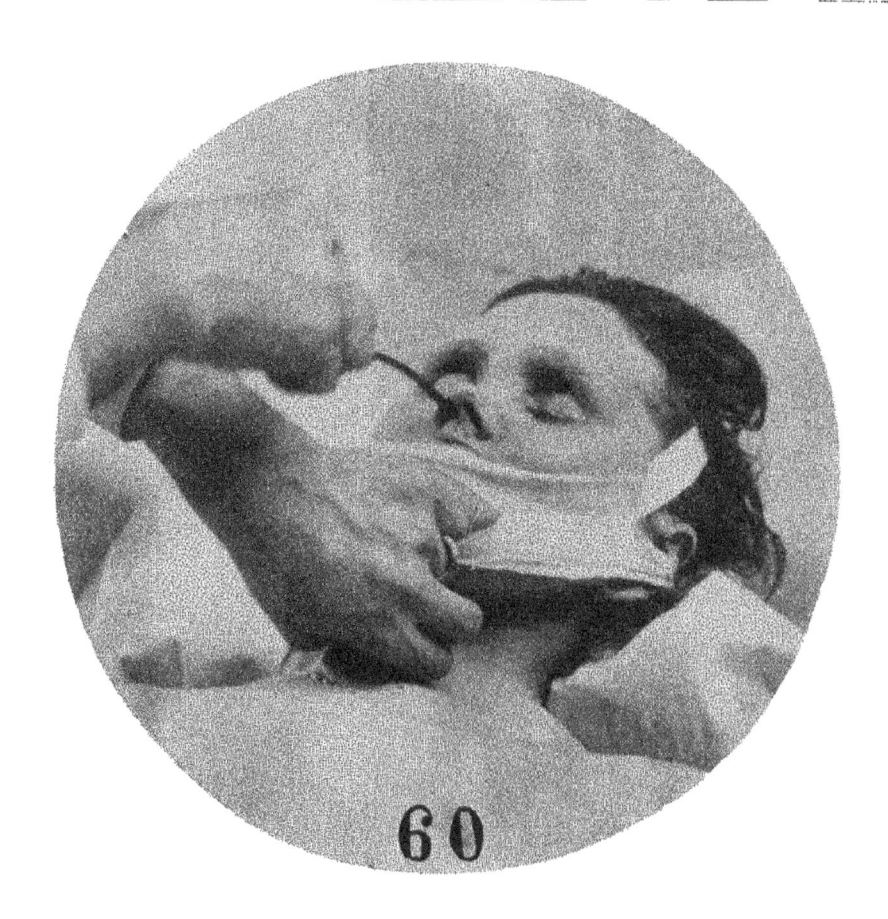

## TO INJECT THE LUNGS THROUGH THE NASAL PASSAGE.

Take the nasal tube and if it is not the proper curvature warm it and bend it to the desired curvature (as per cut No. 59).

Pass it down through the nostril, and allow the fluid to pass through the windpipe, into the lungs, grasp the larynx or Adam's Apple and pull it forward and upward to raise the epiglottis. Then point the nasal tube forward and toward that point, entering the windpipe (as per cut). Then inject Espy's Embalming Fluid.

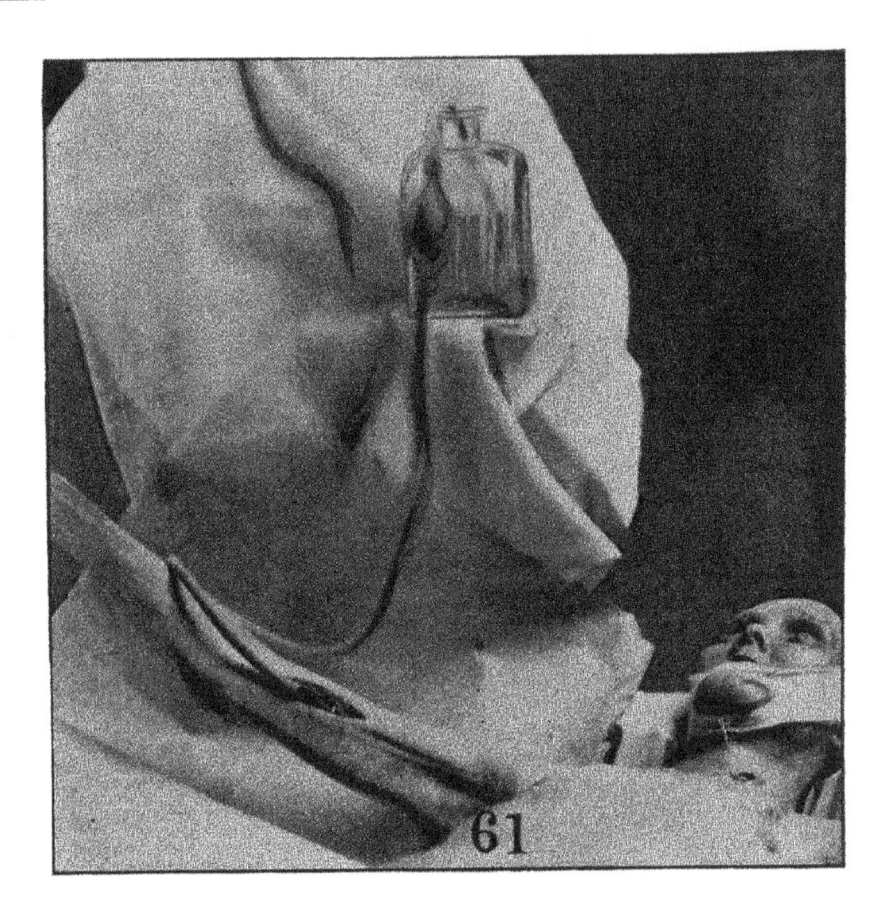

## TO EMBALM A CONSUMPTIVE ARTERIALLY.

Raise the brachial or radial artery and place tube in the artery, per instructions in another place. Now raise the arm above the body, and attach to the arterial tube, either the bulb injector or the syringe. Then take a bottle of fluid and place it on a stand higher than the body. Now place the bulb injector or syringe in the bottle (as per cut), and *very slowly* make one bulb injection just to start the fluid. Then allow the instrument to act as a syphon, the fluid going in by gravitation, and filling the whole vascular system. This will take a little longer, but will not rupture any of the arteries or veins in the lungs. Or you may take a fountain bag, and attaching the tube of it to the arterial tube, place the fluid in the bag, hang the bag above the body and allow the fluid to enter by gravitation. If at any time, while injecting a body arterially, you should rupture any of the arteries or veins in the lungs, and the fluid should run out at the mouth, take a piece of absorbent cotton, and plug the throat. Then take about one tablespoonful of plaster of paris and mix it with water, making a solution of about the thickness of cream, and pour it on the cotton. It will soon harden and you can proceed with your injection.

## Letting off Gasses and Destroying the Odor.

Take a piece of rubber tubing and the trocar and attach one end of the tubing to the trocar. Then take a bottle about one-third full of fluid and place the other end of the tubing in it. Next enter the cavity (as per cuts No. 54, 55, 56 and 57), and allow the gases to pass off through the fluid.

If the stomach and intestines should be distended with gases, make a puncture per instructions elsewhere given, and allow the gases to pass off through the fluid, which will destroy all odor.

## To Puncture the Intestines and Let off the Gases.

Take the trocar and enter the abdominal cavity (as per cut No. 57). Take hold of the trocar with your right hand, and gather up the intestines with your left hand and puncture on the right side. Take the left side in the same way. Then point the trocar upward and toward the left side, and you may puncture the stomach, allowing the gases to pass off, per instructions given in another place.

## To Empty the Stomach.

Turn the body on the right side, while laying level on the board. With the left hand hold the head in position, but do not let it get below the level of the body, for if that is done, the blood will rush to the head and do more damage than good. Then place the right knee in the space just below the ribs on the upper and inner left side, and the right hand on the outer left side. Press with the knee and pull forward with the right hand. This will cause the contents of the stomach to run out at the mouth. Then inject some fluid, through the nasal tube, into the stomach.

## To Thoroughly Embalm a Body.

There is only one way to properly embalm a body, and that is as follows: First draw the blood by instructions given elsewhere. Should there be any gases in any of the cavities, allow them to escape, (per instructions in another place). If there should be any gases in the stomach or intestines, make a puncture with the trocar (per instructions). If not successful in pnucturing the stomach and intestines with the trocar, the last resort is to take the scalpel and make an incision, on the left side of the navel, into the abdominal cavity. Then take the scalpel and puncture the intestines and stomach. After having done that take a sponge and wash the edges of the incision with the fluid. This will tend to close up any arteries or veins you have severed. Then sew the incision up tightly.

This being done, inject the arterial and venous systems, with Espy's Embalming Fluid, through any of the arteries mentioned, always exercising care not to inject the fluid too rapidly, for in so doing, there is great danger of flushing the face, especially if the blood has not all been drawn. The arteries of an adult usually require about two quarts of fluid. If it is certain that circulation is complete it is not always necessary to inject the cavities, but in order to be on the safe side, always inject some fluid into the cavities. It can do no harm, and may do a great deal of good, especially in cases where the disease was in the cavity.

It is sometimes necessary, in very bad cases, to inject a body the second time; but this is seldom the case where Espy's Embalming Fluid has been used. After having finished embalming a body, always sew up the incision neatly.

## To Close the Eyes.

Take a tooth-pick or small sliver, and put a very small bit of cotton on the point of it. Lift the upper lid and place the cotton on the eye-ball; bring the lid down to its place and withdraw the toothpick, leaving the cotton. Hold the lid down and it will then stay. If necessary, bring up the lower lid first, in the same way.

A piece of newspaper, or soft piece of cotton cloth will answer the purpose, instead of the cotton; or, by washing the eyeball off, with the fluid, and pulling the lid down, the eye will remain closed.

## To Close the Mouth.

Take a small piece of cloth and wipe the teeth and gums. Then take about one tablespoonful of plaster of paris and mix it with water, making a solution about the thickness of cream and pour it into the mouth, allowing the solution to run around the teeth and gums. It will soon harden and keep the mouth closed.

## How to Bleach (When Necessary.)

⚜

Take a small, flat camel's hair brush (about an inch and a half wide), and paint the face, ears, neck, hands and all exposed skin with bleacher or diluted fluid. Then place cotton lintine or cloths dampened with the bleacher or diluted fluid on the face and neck, but not on the hands, unless they are very dark. After the animal heat has left the body, it will not be necessary to paint or change the cloths oftener than once in twelve hours.

## Contagious Diseases.

⚜

The first thing to do in case of a contagious disease is for the embalmer disinfect himself, by spraying or sprinkling his clothing hair and beard with Espy's Sure Disinfectant (which is non-poisonous). Then wet the hands in the disinfectant or embalming fluid.

Use at least ten per cent. of the disinfectant or fluid, in the water used to wash the body. After having washed the body, sponge it thoroughly with either the disinfectant or fluid; also spray the hair and beard. Dip some cotton in the disinfectant or fluid and fill the rectum with it. If the subject is a lady, take a large bunch of cotton dipped in the fluid or disinfectant and place it close up against the valva, inside the diaper. Now lay the body on the board at an incline. In these cases *always* inject the whole vascular system. If a full circulation is not assured inject the cavities also. By following these directions, there will be no danger of contagion from the body.

There will be no danger in holding a public funeral, at a church or at the house, provided it has been thoroughly fumigated. The best way to fumigate is to take Espy's Sure Disinfectant, which is odorless and harmless to the person using it. Put it full strength into some old vessel, place it on a stove and let it boil, allowing the steam to penetrate the house or room thoroughly. Have the house or room closed as tightly as possible. Keeping a sponge wet with the disinfectant, suspended in a sick room will prevent the spread of the disease. Use it also in the vessels that are used about the sick person.

## Cancer Cases.

Clean out the cancer, getting all of the corrupt matter out, down to the sound flesh. Then wash it well with the fluid. This will close (to a certain extent), the ends of the arteries and veins. Sprinkle the sore lightly with dry plaster of paris. Now add a thick solution of plaster of paris (which is made by dissolving the plaster of paris in water), until you have the cavity filled. If the cancer is on the face or any exposed part of the body, build it up a little higher and let it harden. Now take the scalpel or a sharp knife, and shave it down to where wanted. Next take some fine sand-paper and smooth it. Then color it a flesh tint and coat it with white shellac, cut in alcohol, giving it several coats until it forms a skin; when dry, rub it with vaseline until it appears like the natural skin. This can be done so that the subject will look very natural. After this, inject both the arteries and cavities.

## A Dropsical Case.

In a dropsical case, draw the water from the cavity (or cavities), by using the aspirator. Then tap the legs at the ankles, and wrap them with strips of muslin or a rubber bandage, commencing at the hips and wrapping down to the ankle. Next wrap the feet, commencing at the toes and wrapping up to the ankles. Tap the body on each side (down close to the board), at the hips, just where the wrapping was commenced. Now wrap the body, commencing above the water, and wrap down to the places tapped. If there is any bloat or water about the hands and arms, tap on the back of the arm at the shoulder joint. Then commence at the tips of the fingers and wrap up to the shoulder. Draw the arms at the elbows well up onto the body. Always have the body on a rubber blanket, and at an incline. *Always* inject the arterial system, together with the cavities. Sometimes it is necessary to inject the body two or three times at about twelve hour intervals. In such cases always leave the arterial tube in the artery until the last injecton. Do not rub the face or hands, as there is danger of the skin slipping. By following these instructions no trouble should be experienced.

## How to Take Care of a Floater.

If you have a *very* bad case of this kind, the best way to take care of it is to *bury* it. If it has not been in the water very long, and it is desired to keep it for a few days or ship it, follow the directions below.

When the body is taken out of the water, lay it face downward on a barrel, and roll it and get all the water out possible. Use the femoral vein tube in the femoral vein, in connection with the brachial or radial artery, per instructions given elsewhere. Eject (or aspirate), and inject alternately (per instructions with cut No. 52), until the embalming fluid makes its appearance. Always keep the body at an incline. Rub the face and neck downward and use the hot water applications, if necessary. Also empty the cavities of water and then inject them with fluid. In these cases it is sometimes necessary to inject the body two or three times at about twelve hour intervals; but in cases where the tissues are broken down, all that can be done is to inject the cavities with a VERY STRONG fluid, to arrest decomposition for a short time. Espy's Quadruple Strength will do this.

# To Embalm Cases Where Death was Caused by Diseases of the Abdominal Cavity (Such as Peritonitis, Child-Birth, Inflammation of the Bowels, &c.)

First let off the gases, by instructions in previous chapters. Then attach the aspirator to the trocar and place it in an empty bottle. Next attach the drawing side of the pump to the aspirator and then aspirate all the matter that you can get. If the matter is too thick to be drawn through the trocar, insert another trocar into the abdominal cavity. Both trocars should be just below the navel, one on each side. Now attach another aspirator or injector to the trocar last inserted, and place it in a bottle full of fluid. Next attach the injecting side of the pump to this aspirator or injector. Then begin to pump, which injects fluid and aspirates or draws matter at the same time (as per cut No. 52); the fluid thinning the matter. Or you may inject and aspirate alternately, until you have washed all the matter from the cavity. Now fill the cavity with fluid and then remove the trocars, closing the incisions with drawstrings, as per instructions elsewhere.

Another way to treat cases of this kind is to make an incision below the navel, about three inches long. Next take a sponge and wash all the matter out of the cavity. Fill the cavity with fluid and sew up the incision. It is always best to draw the blood in these cases, for the blood gives us more trouble than any other matter of the body. In these cases, always inject the whole vascular system. In bad cases leave the arterial tube in the artery until after you have injected the last time, placing a closed-end thimble over same to prevent leakage. In about eighteen hours inject more fluid.

## Double Pneumonia.

First wash all the corruption from both lung cavities, by using two trocars, an aspirator's pump and injector, per instructions given for cleansing the abdominal cavity; cleansing first one lung and then the other. Now fill both the cavities with the fluid. In these cases always inject the arterial system, together with the lung cavities; but do not use too much fluid at the first injection. Leave the arterial tube in the artery, and in from eight to twelve hours go back and inject the body again.

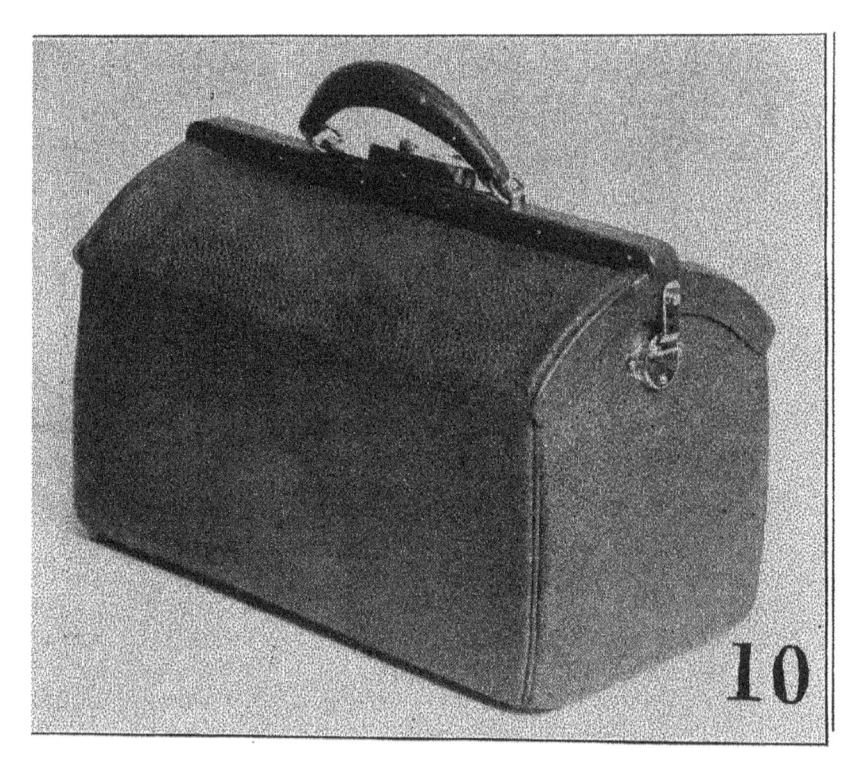

ESPY'S NEW CABINET GRIP.

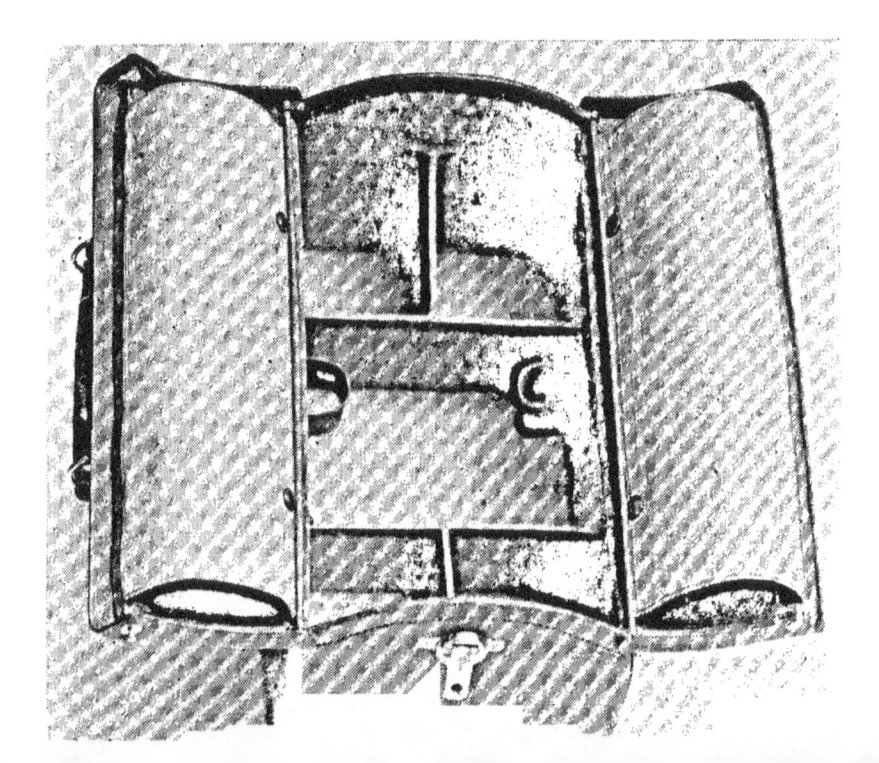

ESPY'S EMBALMER. 77

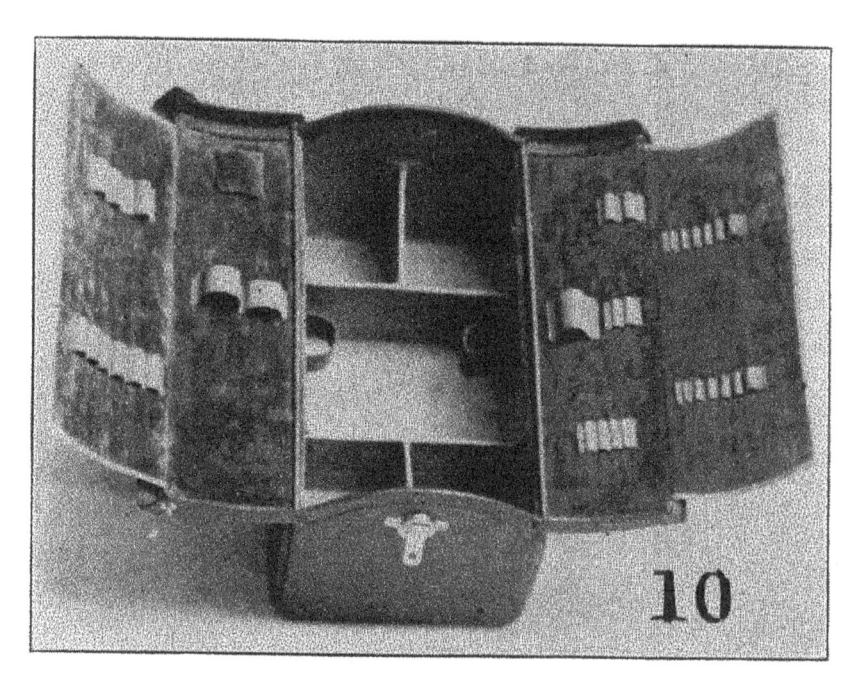

ESPY'S NEW CABINET GRIP, OPEN. PRICE, $10.00.

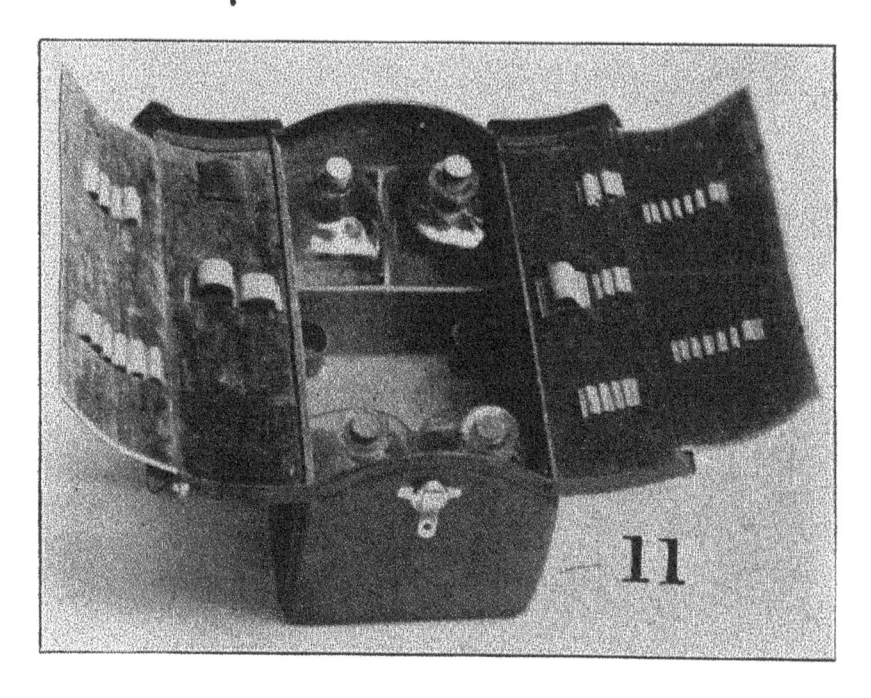

ESPYS NEW CABINET GRIP WITH BOTTLES. PRICE, $11.00.

78 ESPY'S EMBALMER.

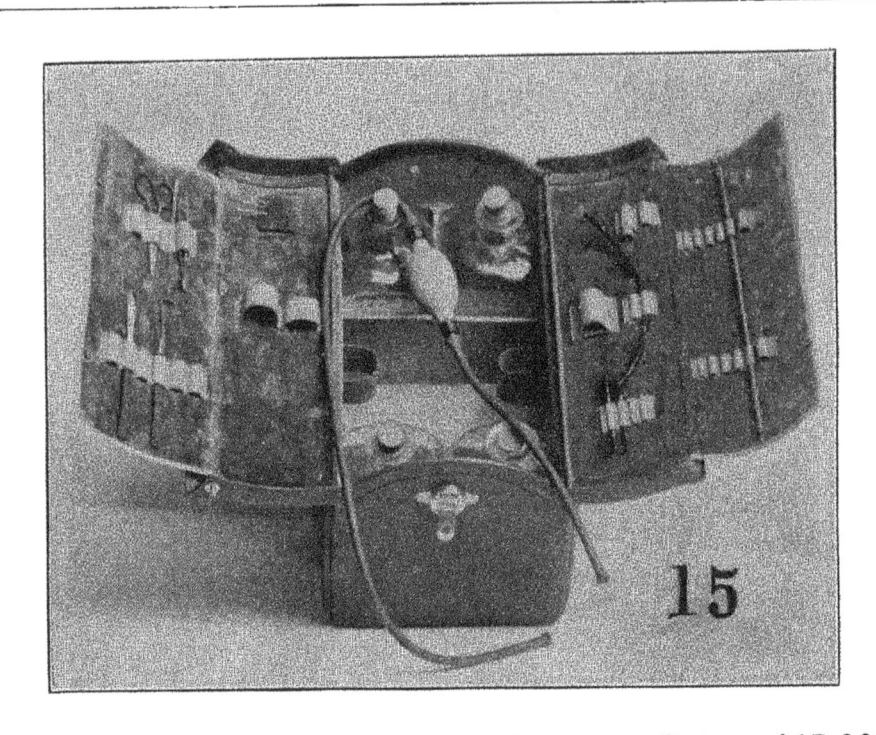

## Espy's New Cabinet Grip, No. 15.  Price, $15.00.
### CONTAINING:

| | | |
|---|---|---|
| 1 | Syringe.................................................. | $ 2 00 |
| 2 | Arterial Tubes........................................ | 50 |
| 1 | Trocar................................................... | 1 50 |
| 1 | Scalpel.................................................. | 75 |
| 1 | Aneurism Needle................................... | 75 |
| 1 | pair Forceps.......................................... | 75 |
| 1 | pair Scissors.......................................... | 75 |
| 1 | Hard Rubber Nasal Tube....................... | 75 |
| 1 | Flexible Catheter................................... | 25 |
| 1 | Closed-end Thimble............................... | 05 |
| 1 | Fascia Needle........................................ | 25 |
| 3 | Surgeons' Needles................................. | 15 |
| 4 | Empty Quart Bottles and Stoppers......... | 1 00 |
| 1 | Cabinet Grip.......................................... | 10 00 |

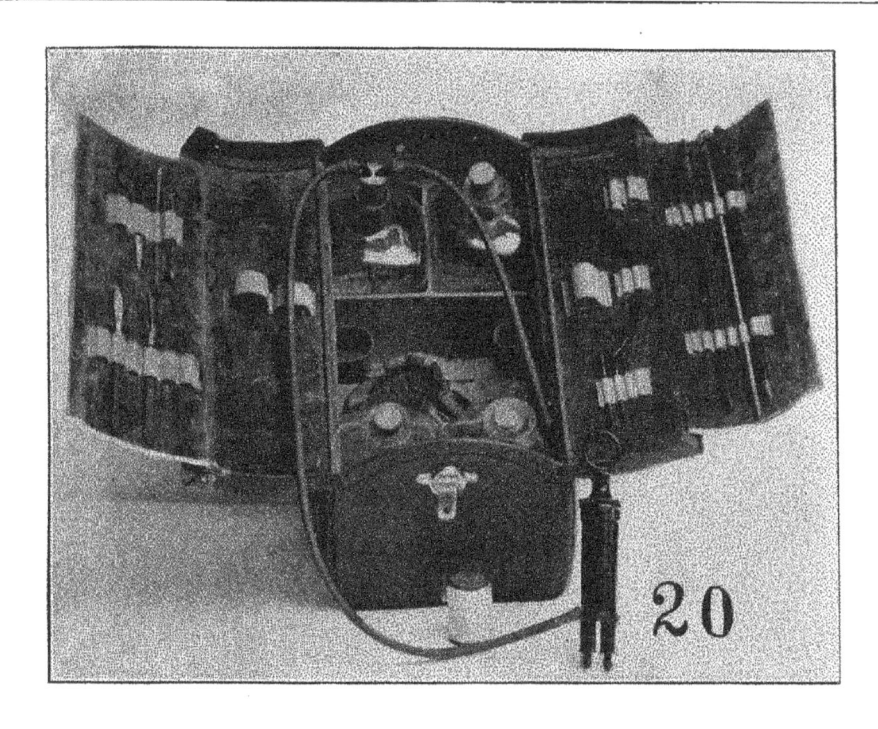

## Espy's New Cabinet Grip, No. 20.   Price, $20.00.
### CONTAINING:

| | | |
|---|---|---|
| 1 | Hard Rubber Pump................................. | $ 4 00 |
| 1 | Aspirator .......................................... | 1 00 |
| 3 | Arterial Tubes..................................... | 75 |
| 2 | Trocars............................................ | 3 00 |
|   | Scalpel............................................ | 75 |
|   | Aneurism Needle................................... | 75 |
|   | pair Forceps....................................... | 75 |
|   | pair Scissors....................................... | 75 |
|   | Hard Rubber Nasal Tube........................... | 75 |
| 1 | Flexible Catheter.................................. | 25 |
|   | Closed-end Thimble................................ | 05 |
|   | Fascia Needle...................................... | 25 |
| 3 | Surgeons' Needles ................................. | 15 |
| 1 | Spool Linen Thread and Wax....................... | 10 |
| 1 | Sponge and Rubber Bag............................ | 35 |
| 4 | Empty Quart Bottles and Stoppers.................. | 1 00 |
| 1 | Cabinet Grip...................................... | 10 00 |

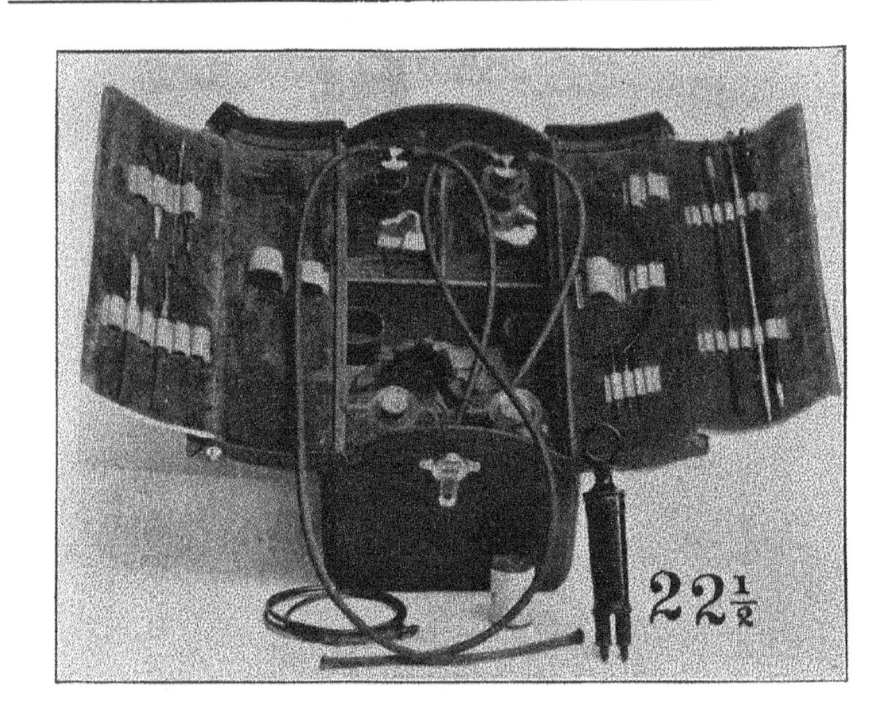

## Espy's New Cabinet Grip, No. 22½. Price, $22.50.

### CONTAINING:

| | | |
|---|---|---|
| 1 | Hard Rubber Pump............................................. | $ 4 00 |
| 2 | Aspirators.......................................................... | 2 00 |
| 3 | Arterial Tubes................................................... | 75 |
| 2 | Trocars.............................................................. | 3 00 |
|   | Scalpel................................................................ | 75 |
|   | Aneurism Needle................................................. | 75 |
|   | pair Forceps........................................................ | 75 |
|   | pair Scissors....................................................... | 75 |
|   | Hard Rubber Nasal Tube..................................... | 75 |
| 1 | Flexible Catheter................................................. | 25 |
|   | Femoral Vein Tube............................................... | 2 50 |
|   | Closed-end Thimble............................................. | 05 |
| 1 | Fascia Needle...................................................... | 25 |
| 3 | Surgeons' Needles............................................... | 15 |
| 1 | Spool Linen Thread and Wax............................... | 10 |
| 1 | Sponge and Rubber Bag...................................... | 35 |
| 4 | Empty Quart Bottles and Stoppers........................ | 1 00 |
| 1 | Cabinet Grip........................................................ | 10 00 |

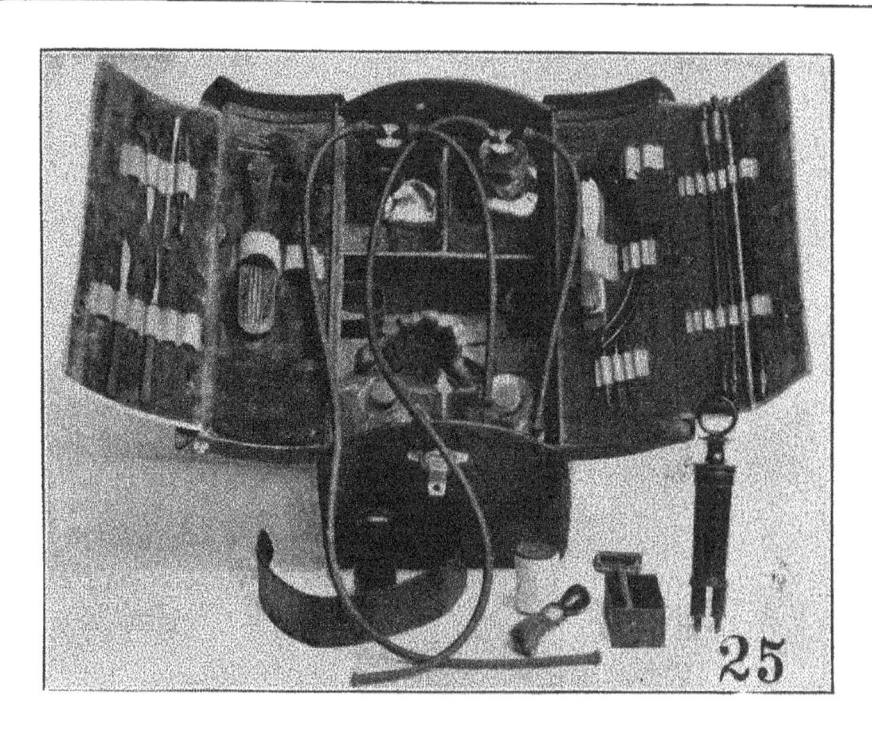

## Espy's New Cabinet Grip, No. 25.   Price, $25.00.
### CONTAINING:

| | |
|---|---:|
| 1 Hard Rubber Pump | $ 4 00 |
| 2 Aspirators | 2 00 |
| 3 Arterial Tubes | 75 |
| 2 Trocars | 3 00 |
| 1 Scalpel | 75 |
| 1 Aneurism Needle | 75 |
| 1 pair Forceps | 75 |
| 1 pair Scissors | 75 |
| 2 Nasal Tubes | 1 50 |
| 2 Catheters | 50 |
| 2 Closed-end Thimbles | 10 |
| 1 Fascia Needle | 25 |
| 3 Surgeon's Needles | 15 |
| 1 Spool of Thread and Wax | 10 |
| 1 Safety or Handle Razor | 2 00 |
| 1 Razor Strop | 50 |
| 1 Shaving Brush | 25 |
| 1 Comb | 10 |
| 1 Hair Brush | 25 |
| 1 Stick of Shaving Soap | 25 |
| 1 Nail Brush | 25 |
| 1 Rubber Bag and Sponge | 35 |
| 4 Empty Quart Bottles and Stoppers | 1 00 |
| 1 Cabinet Grip | 10 00 |

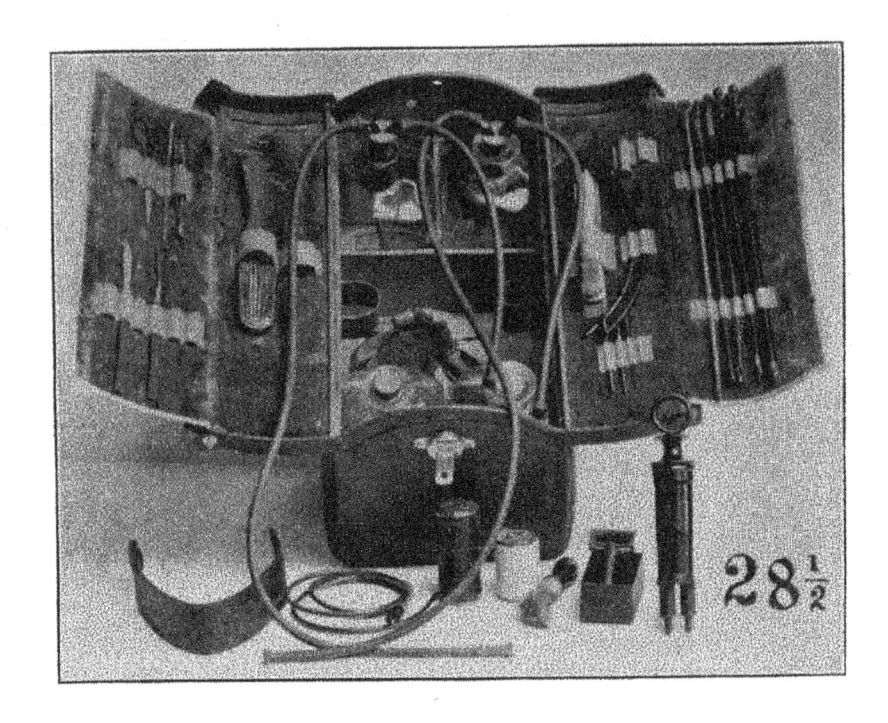

## Espy's New Cabinet Grip, No. 28½.  Price, $28.50.
### CONTAINING:

| | |
|---|---:|
| 1 Hard Rubber Pump | $ 4 00 |
| 2 Aspirators | 2 00 |
| 3 Arterial Tubes | 75 |
| 2 Trocars | 3 00 |
| 1 Dropsical Trocar | 2 00 |
| 1 Scalpel | 75 |
| 1 Anuerism Needle | 75 |
| 1 pair Forceps | 75 |
| 1 pair Scissors | 75 |
| 2 Nasal Tubes | 1 50 |
| 2 Catheters | 50 |
| 2 Closed-end Thimbles | 10 |
| 1 Fascia Needle | 25 |
| 3 Surgeons' Needles | 15 |
| 1 Spool of Thread and Wax | 10 |
| 1 Safety or Handle Razor | 2 00 |
| 1 Razor Strop | 50 |
| 1 Shaving Brush | 25 |
| 1 Comb | 10 |
| 1 Hair Brush | 25 |
| 1 Stick of Shaving Soap | 25 |
| 1 Nail Brush | 25 |
| 1 Rubber Bag and Sponge | 35 |
| 1 Femoral Vein Tube | 2 50 |
| 4 Empty Quart Bottles and Stoppers | 1 00 |
| 1 Cabinet Grip | 10 00 |

## Espy's New Cabinet Grip.

This is the most complete Embalmers' Grip, for the price, that is on the market today.

It has the round frame, which adds to its beauty as well as to its capacity. It is also provided with inside flaps or covers, which protect the instruments from dampness and which are fastened to the outer edge of the frame, so as to open out instead of in, thereby giving the embalmer access to the inside of the Grip without interference. These flaps or covers are provided with loops for the longer instruments (as the Trocars and Catheters), so that they may be placed in position or withdrawn without the usual obstruction that is met with in the old style grips.

Our Grip is designed to carry four quart bottles and is provided with sufficient loops to carry all the instruments that would be required by the most expert embalmer. It presents a very neat appearance and is very compact, every inch of space being utilized. The workmanship is of the BEST, as well as the material used in its construction.

If you contemplate buying a Grip, you will regret it if you make your purchase before seeing and examining ours.

**STEEL TROCARS.**—Just a word about our Steel Trocars. It is quite natural for us to think that we have the BEST; but we will not say anything about that, and let you decide for yourself. All we ask is for you to give them a trial. We have them in all sizes made of solid drawn steel, highly tempered. We guarantee them to be of SUPERIOR QUALITY.

**HARD RUBBER TROCARS.**—You will kindly pardon us for saying a word about our Hard Rubber Trocars. The points are made of highly tempered steel, heavily nickel plated. The rubber is vulcanized on the point in such a manner as to make it impossible to break them where the rubber joins the steel. The steel rod on the inside is coated with hard rubber, to make it proof against corroding. By this we overcome the difficulty that is to be contended with in using the steel rod, which so often corrodes and sticks to the point.

**OUR HARD RUBBER DROPSICAL TROCAR** supplies a long-felt want. It is made of hard rubber, as described above, and is provided with a diamond-shaped point, the three sides of which are milled out in such a way as to admit the water from the point of the trocar. Thus you are enabled to draw all the water from the body; while in the old style trocar the holes or slots are an inch or two up from the point, and you cannot draw the water after you get down to the top of the holes or slots. "A word to the wise is sufficient." In ordering please mention number and prices.

MANUFACTURED BY
THE ESPY FLUID CO., SPRINGFIELD, O.

## Espy's Rubber Pillows.

Designed to take the place of the old style, hard head rest. Can be used on any cooling-board. Made in two sizes.

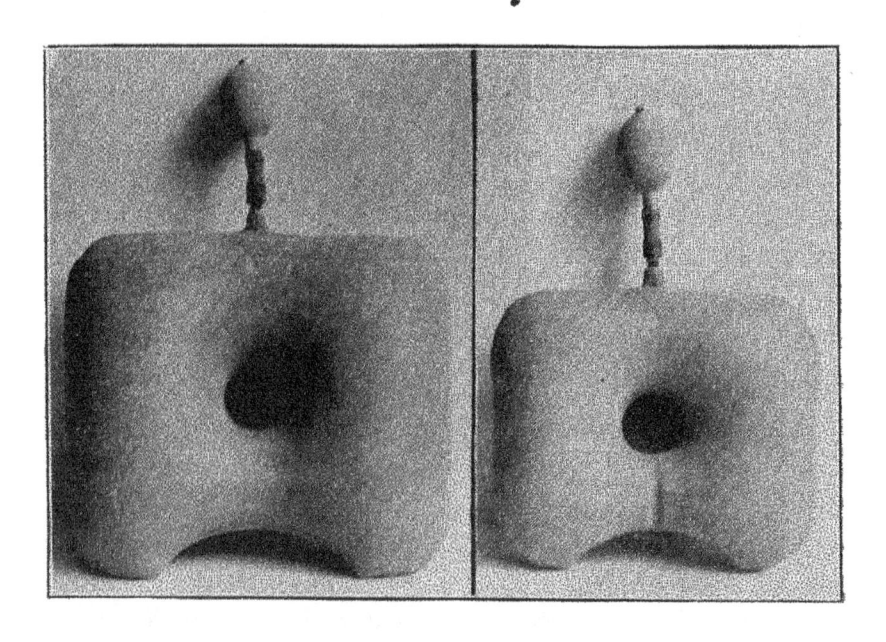

LARGE SIZE. Price, $2.50.   MEDIUM. Price, $2.00.

MANUFACTURED BY
THE ESPY FLUID CO., SPRINGFIELD, O.

ER.    85

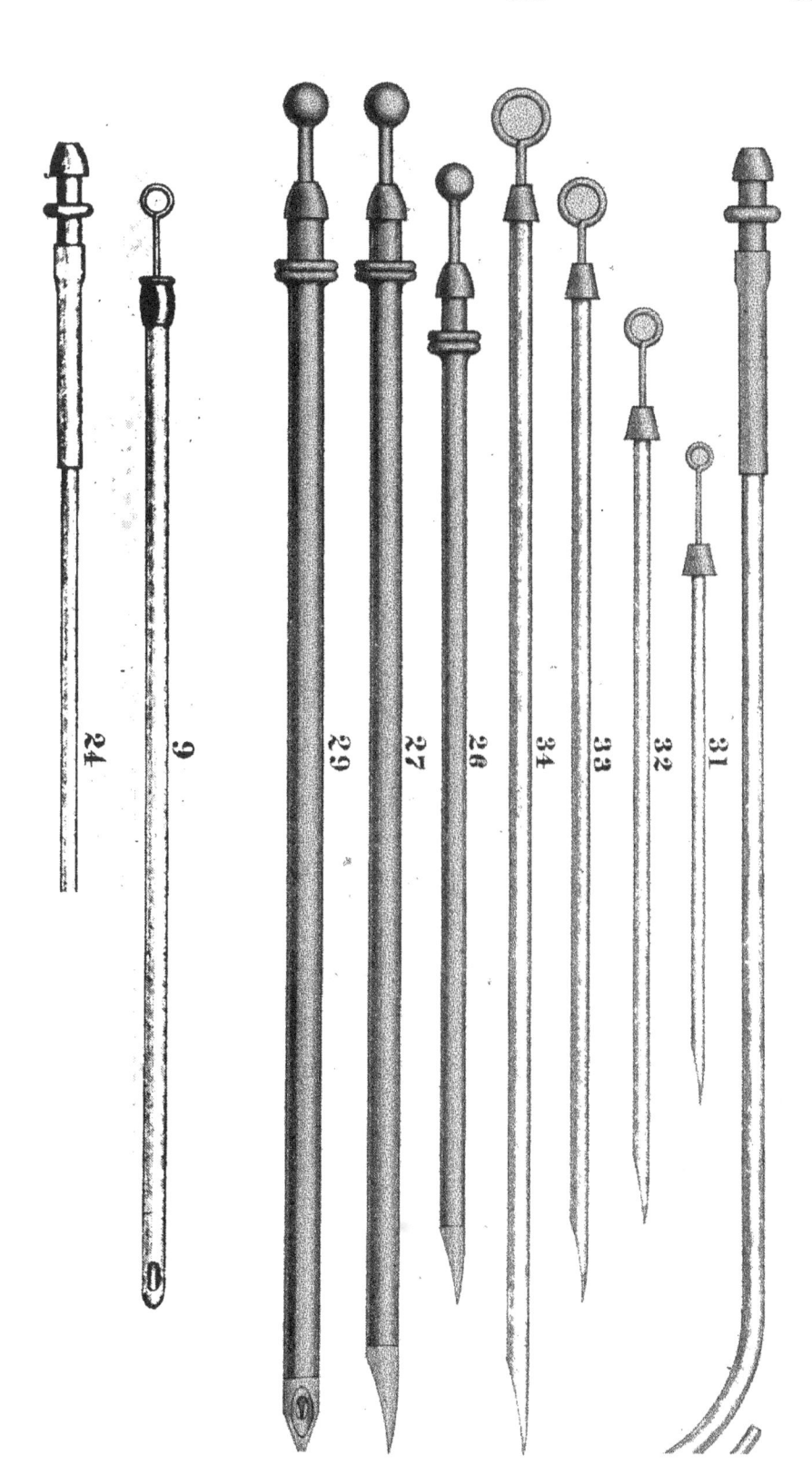

# Espy's New Hard Rubber Pump Aspirator and Injector.

Espy's New Hard Rubber Pump is made by skilled workmen and of the very best rubber. It possesses ALL the requirements of a first-class embalmer's pump.

THE VALVES ARE VERY SENSITIVE, as well as strong and durable, and are much superior to the old style valve. The least movement of the piston brings the pump into action at once, and it works smoothly from one end of the cylinder to the other. There is no lost motion with which to contend, as the valves are self-acting.

THE SUCKERS on the piston rod are the new, improved ones, packed with a material that retains the oil and keeps them soft and pliable for an indefinite length of time.

OUR TUBING is of the very best that can be made. It is provided with the rolled ends, which make it neat and attractive in appearance. It is strong and durable, easy to connect with the arterial tube or trocar, and when connected is air-tight and will not leak.

THE ROLLED-END TUBING costs us considerably more than the ordinary kind, but it is our highest ambition to give our customers the best that can be produced, regardless of cost.

The Espy Pump is a combined aspirator or injector. It can be used either to inject or aspirate, or you can inject and aspirate at the same time, as occasion may require. Directions accompany each Pump, fully explaining how to aspirate. Cut and prices will be found on another page.

MANUFACTURED BY

*THE ESPY FLUID CO.*, SPRINGFIELD, O.

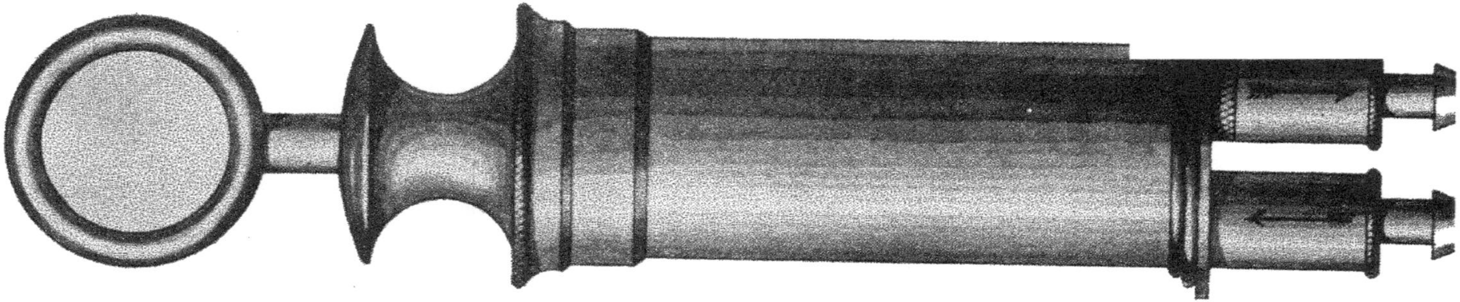

## PRICE OF ESPY'S NEW HARD RUBBER PUMP.

*Manufactured by* **THE ESPY FLUID CO., Springfield, O.**

| | |
|---|---|
| Pump | $ 4 00 |
| Pump with three Arterial Tubes | 4 75 |
| Pump with three Arterial Tubes and one Aspirator | 5 75 |
| Pump with three Arterial Tubes and two Aspirators | 6 75 |

**COMPLETE DIRECTIONS ACCOMPANYING EACH.**

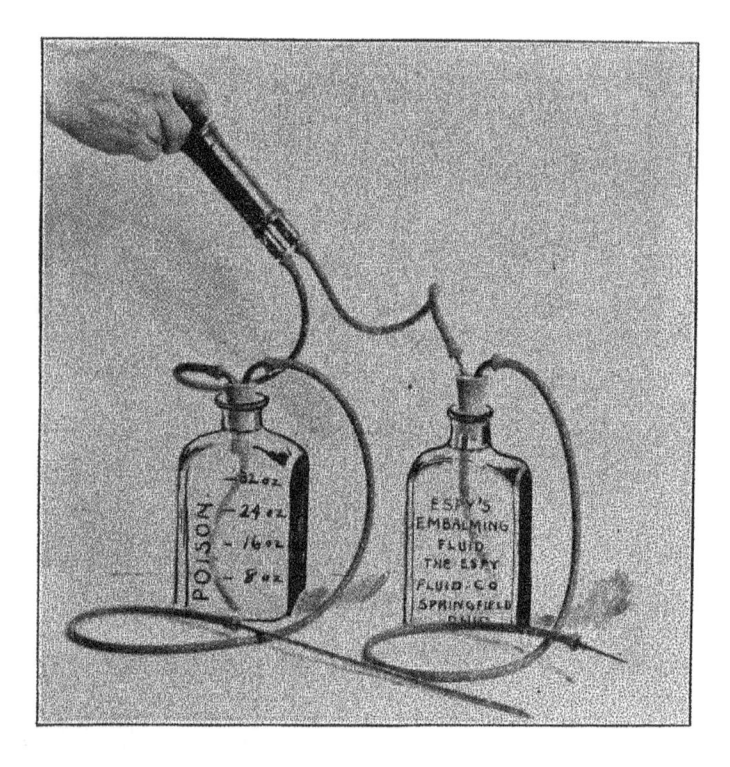

*The Above Cut Shows the Pump in Position for Injecting and Ejecting.*

## DRAINING TUBES.

For drawing the blood from the body through the Basilic and Femoral veins. Made of silk and coated with rubber.

Basilic vein tube, 24 inches long, each................ ....$1 25
Femoral vein tube, 36 inches long, each................. 2 50

The latest improved Safety Razor, each.................... 2 00
A good Handle Razor, each............................... 2 00

## SURGEONS' NEEDLES.

Each, 5c, or 25 cents per half dozen.

---

MANUFACTURED BY AND FOR

*THE ESPY FLUID CO.*, SPRINGFIELD, O.

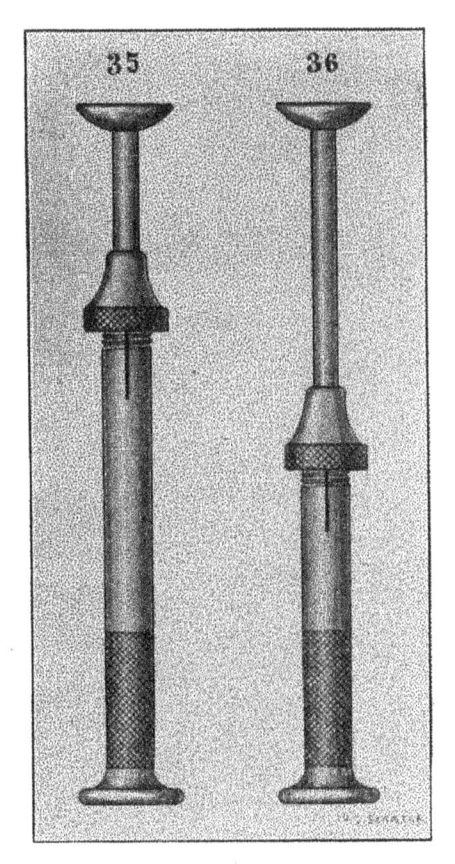

## ESPY'S HARD RUBBER ADJUSTABLE CHIN SUPPORT,

Our new Hard Rubber Chin Support is an article that will be appreciated by the up-to-date embalmer. It is made of the best hard rubber and in a neat, substantial manner. It can be adjusted to any desired length. It will not corrode and is always clean and presentable. Made in two sizes.

No. 35. Price, each................................... 40c
No. 36. Price, each................................... 40c
The two for .............................................. 75c

## ESPY'S BULB SYRINGE.

With Hard Rubber Fittings and the best of Tubing, complete.
No. 52. Price ...................................................$2 00

If you are needing anything in our line, send us your order and it will receive our prompt attention.

**THE ESPY FLUID CO., SPRINGFIELD, O.**

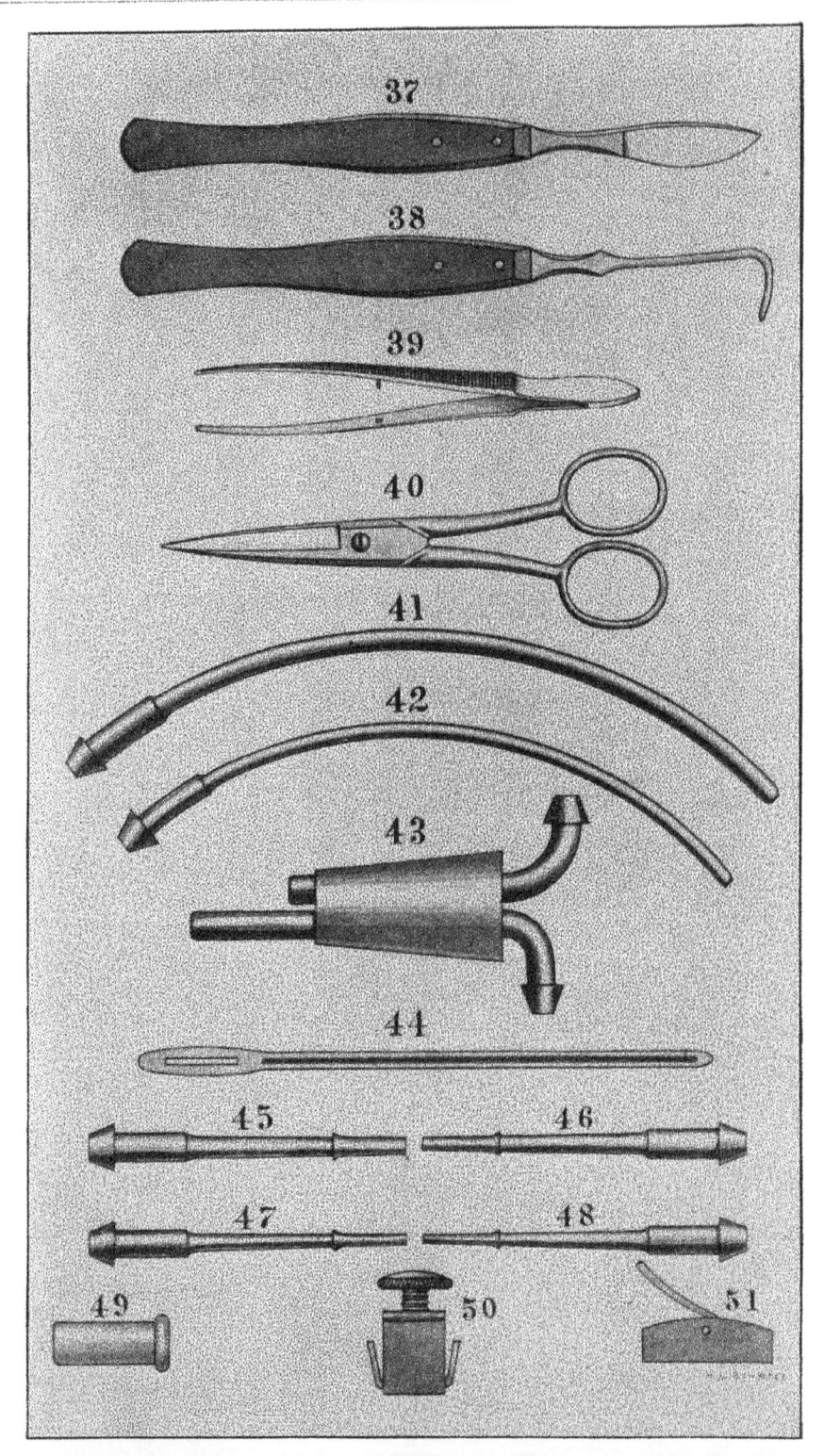

INSTRUMENTS MANUFACTURED BY THE ESPY FLUID CO.

# Price List of Instruments Manufactured by the Espy Fluid Co.

Espy's New Cabinet Grip. No. 10, empty............................................$10 00
Espy's New Cabinet Grip, No. 11, with bottles ....................... 11 00
Espy's New Cabinet Grip, No. 15, with instruments (as per cut). 15 00
Espy's New Cabinet Grip, No. 20, with instruments (as per cut), 20 00
Espy's New Cabinet Grip, No. 22½, with instruments (as per cut), 22 50
Espy's New Cabinet Grip, No. 25, with instruments (as per cut), 25 00
Espy's New Cabinet Grip, No. 28½, with instruments (as per cut), 28 50
   See cuts of Grips and Instruments elsewhere.

| No. | Item | Price |
|---|---|---|
| No. 1. | Espy's Hard Rubber Pump | 4 00 |
| No. 52. | Bulb Syringe, with Hard Rubber Fittings | 2 00 |
| No. 43. | Aspirator | 1 00 |
| No. 45, 46, 47, 48. | Arterial Tubes, each | 25 |
| No. 31. | 5-inch Steel Trocar | 75 |
| No. 32. | 7½-inch Steel Trocar | 1 00 |
| No. 33. | 10-inch Steel Trocar | 1 50 |
| No. 34. | 12-inch Steel Trocar | 1 50 |
| No. 26. | 10-inch Hard Rubber Trocar | 1 50 |
| No. 27. | 12-inch Hard Rubber Trocar | 1 50 |
| No. 29. | 12-inch Hard Rubber Dropsical Trocar | 2 00 |
| No. 37. | Scalpel | 75 |
| No. 38. | Aneurism Needle | 75 |
| No. 39. | Forceps | 75 |
| No. 40. | Scissors | 75 |
| No. 41. | Nasal Tube (large size) | 75 |
| No. 42. | Nasal Tube (small size) | 75 |
| No. 9. | Catheter | 25 |
| No. 12. | Catheter | 25 |
| No. 44. | Fascia Needle | 25 |
| No. 49. | Closed-end Soft Rubber Thimble | 05 |
| No. 24. | Basilic Vein Tube | 1 25 |
| No. 23. | Femoral Vein Tube | 2 50 |
| No. 51. | Hard Rubber Cut-off | 25 |
| No. 50. | Graduating Hard Rubber Cut-off | 25 |
| No. 35. | Adjustable Hard Rubber Chin Support (small size) | 40 |
| No. 36. | Adjustable Hard Rubber Chin Support (large size) | 40 |
|  | Espy's Quart Bottle with Stopper | 25 |
|  | New Style Rolled-end Tubing. 12 inches long | 15 |
|  | New Style Rolled-end Tubing. 28 inches long | 25 |
|  | New Style Rolled-end Tubing. 40 inches long | 35 |
|  | Surgeon Needle | 05 |

# Price List of Espy's Embalming Fluid.

| | |
|---|---:|
| 1, 2, 3 and 5 gallons, in jugs, per gallon | $ 2 25 |
| 5 gallons in kegs, per gallon | 2 15 |
| 10 gallons in kegs, per gallon | 2 00 |
| 20 gallons in kegs, per gallon | 1 85 |
| 25 gallons in kegs, per gallon | 1 75 |
| Barrels, containing 48–52 gallons, per gallon | 1 65 |

### ESPY'S QUADRUPLE STRENGTH.—For Cavities.

| | |
|---|---:|
| Per gallon | $ 3 00 |

### ESPY'S POSITIVE BLEACHER.

| | |
|---|---:|
| Pint bottles, per dozen | $ 3 00 |
| 5 gallons, per gallon | 1 00 |

### ESPY'S SURE DISINFECTANT.

| | |
|---|---:|
| Quart bottles, per dozen | $ 6 00 |
| 5 gallons, per gallon | 1 00 |
| 10 gallons, per gallon | 75 |
| Barrels, per gallon | 60 |

*ALL COMPOUNDED AND GUARANTEED BY*

### THE ESPY FLUID CO., SPRINGFIELD, O.

**TERMS.**—All instruments, net 30 days. Fluid, 5 per cent. off 30 days, or net 90 days. Freight on all packages of 10 gallons and upward, to Missouri River.

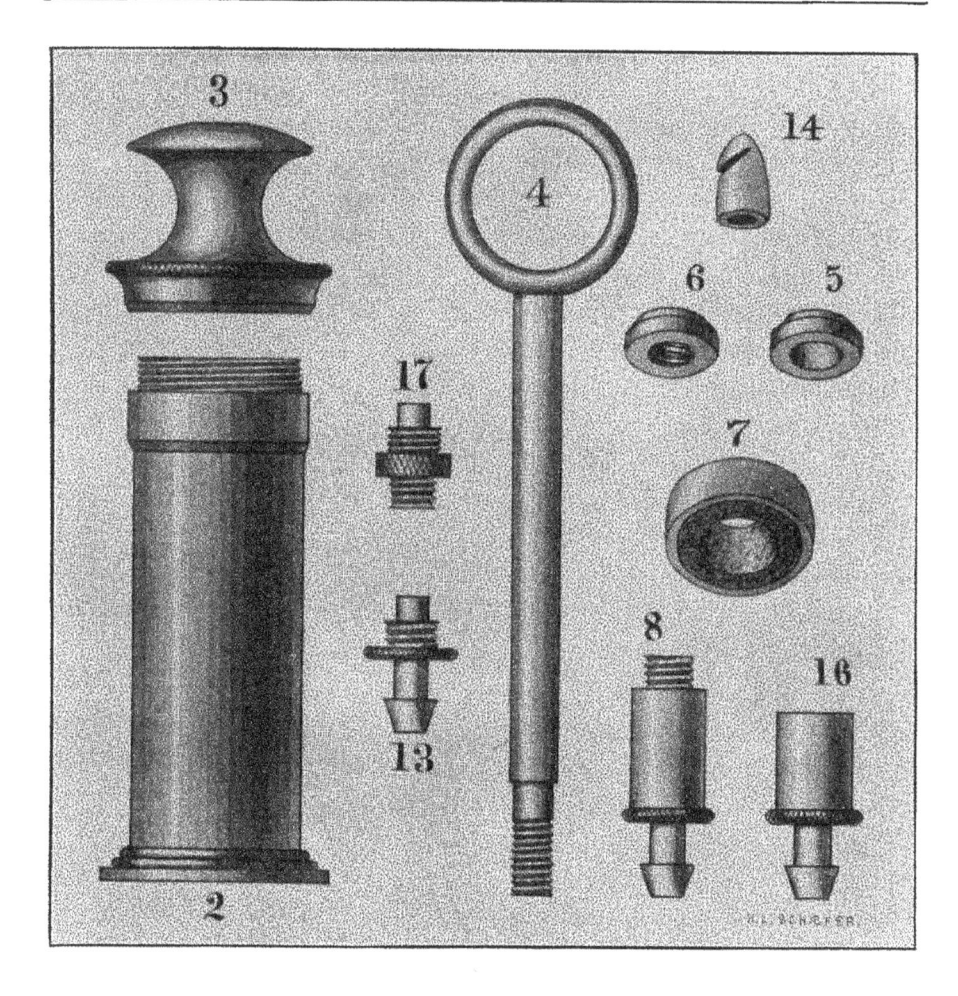

## Price List of Repairs for Espy's Hard Rubber Pump.

| | | | |
|---|---|---|---|
| No. 2. | Barrel | | $ 1 00 |
| No. 3. | Cap | | 75 |
| No. 4. | Piston Rod | | 75 |
| No. 5. | Inner Shoulder on Piston | | 10 |
| No. 6. | Outer Shoulder on Piston | | 10 |
| No. 7. | Leather Suckers, with packing, per pair | | 30 |
| No. 8. | Valve Box with thread on | | 25 |
| No. 16. | Valve box without thread on | | 25 |
| No. 17. | Inner end of Valve Box | | 25 |
| No. 13. | Outer end of Valve Box | | 25 |
| No. 14. | Valve | | 05 |

When ordering repairs please mention the number and price.

**THE ESPY FLUID CO., SPRINGFIELD, O.**

# INDEX.

|  | PAGE. |
|---|---|
| Arteries, Veins and Nerves—How to distinguish | 7 |
| Auricle of the Heart—Tapping the right | 58 |
| Abdominal Cavity—How to inject the | 64 |
| Abdominal Cavity—How to inject | 62 |
| Brachial Artery—How to raise the | 18-27 |
| Basilic Vein—How to locate and raise the | 44-52 |
| Bleach—How to (when necessary) | 72 |
| Brain Cavity—How to inject the | 60 |
| Circulation of the Blood | 5 |
| Circulation of the Fluid in arterial embalming | 6 |
| Carotid Artery, common—How to locate and raise; perpendicular incision | 28-33 |
| Carotid Artery, common—How to raise; transverse incision | 34-38 |
| Cancer Cases | 73 |
| Consumptive—How to embalm; arterially | 68 |
| Dropsical Cases | 73 |
| Double Pneumonia Cases | 75 |
| Draining Tubes, Catheters, Steel and Hard Rubber Trocars | 85 |
| Draining Tubes | 88 |
| Eyes—How to close the | 71 |
| Espy's New Cabinet Grip | 76-83 |
| Espy's Rubber Pillows | 84 |
| Espy's New Hard Rubber Pump | 86-87 |
| Espy's Hard Rubber Chin Support | 89 |
| Espy's Bulb Syringe | 89 |
| Floater—How to take care of a | 74 |
| Femoral Artery—How to locate and raise the | 39-43 |
| Femoral Vein—How to locate and raise the | 53-56 |
| Femoral Vein—Drawing blood from | 56 |
| Gases—How to let off, and destroy the odor | 69 |
| General Instruction | 4 |
| General Price List | 91 |

## INDEX—CONTINUED.

| | PAGE. |
|---|---|
| Heart—Drawing blood from, and draining the body | 59-60 |
| How to thoroughly embalm a body | 70 |
| Intestines—How to puncture, and let off gases | 69 |
| Lungs—How to inject through the nasal passage | 67 |
| Mouth—How to close the | 71 |
| Price List of Espy's Embalming Fluid | 92 |
| Price List of Repairs for Espy's H. R. Pump | 93 |
| Razors | 88 |
| Radial Artery—How to raise the | 8-17 |
| Special Cases—How to treat (such as Peritonitis, Child Birth, Inflammation of the Bowels, etc.) | 75 |
| Surgeon's Needles | 88 |
| Small Instruments | 90 |
| Stomach—How to empty the | 70 |
| Stomach—How to inject through the nasal passage | 66 |
| Thoraci or Lung Cavity—How to inject; by one incision | 61 |
| Thoraci or Lung Cavities—How to inject; by two incisions | 63 |
| Trocar Incision—How to sew up the | 65 |
| Ventricle of the Heart—Tapping the right | 57 |